Con

You.   ¿s

Advisory Editor
Michael Bender, Ed.D.
Vice President of Educational Programs,
The Kennedy Institute;
Professor of Education, The Johns Hopkins University;
Joint Appointment, Department of Pediatrics,
The John Hopkins School of Medicine, Baltimore

Communicable Disease and Young Children in Group Settings

Janeen McCracken Taylor, Ph.D.
The George Washington University,
Washington, D.C.

W. Scott Taylor, M.D.
Sinai Hospital, Baltimore

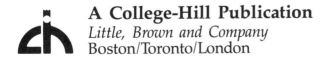

A College-Hill Publication
Little, Brown and Company
Boston/Toronto/London

College-Hill Press
A Division of
Little, Brown and Company (Inc.)
34 Beacon Street
Boston, Massachusetts 02108

Library of Congress Cataloging in Publication Data
Main entry under title:

Taylor, Janeen McCracken, 1946–
    Communicable disease and young children in group settings / by Janeen McCracken Taylor and W. Scott Taylor.
        p.   cm.
    "A College-Hill publication"
    Bibliography: p.
    Includes index.
    ISBN 0-316-83385-1
    1. Communicable diseases in children. 2. Children—health and
hygiene.   I. Taylor, W. Scott (William Scott), 1936–
II. Title.
RJ401.T38   1989   89-2754
618.92 9—dc19   CIP

ISBN 0-316-83385-1

Printed in the United States of America
EB

For
Scott, Douglas, James, Kyra, and Wesley
and
Lt. Col. (USAF, Retired) and Mrs. Robert Lee McCracken

Contents

Preface

My interest in communicable diseases and young children started in the mid-1970s. I was a teacher at a marvelous preschool for young children with handicaps (Albuquerque Special Preschool, now named Alta Mira). In a casual conversation, a mother of an infant enrolled in our program mentioned that her daughter was handicapped as a result of congenital cytomegalovirus (CMV) infection. She had never heard of CMV and was unsure of how it caused her child's developmental delays. I was also unfamiliar with CMV, but knew many colleagues who could share information about this disease. Several of my co-workers were pregnant and concerned about the health and development of their unborn children. County health officials, pediatricians, and obstetricians, including my husband (and co-author) Scott, informed us about CMV. It became evident that inservice education regarding communicable diseases should be an integral part of training for early childhood special educators.

A few years later, and many hundreds of miles away, I was working with the director of special education in Maryland. I was asked to identify emerging issues in early childhood special education. After conducting a literature review and surveying leaders in the field, a number of issues surfaced, among them, communicable diseases. I collaborated with colleagues in the state health department to develop policies and training programs focused on minimizing transmission of communicable diseases in educational settings. This experience increased my awareness of the importance of understanding how communicable diseases are spread in group settings of young children and provided an incentive to explore an area foreign to many teachers. The literature and information gathered over the years serves as the foundation for this text.

As the number of children cared for in out-of-home placements increases, research regarding disease transmission in child care programs is being reported with greater frequency in medical journals. However, relatively few articles in early childhood and special education journals and texts have addressed this timely topic. The writing of this book was undertaken in an attempt to provide a readable guide to current information about communicable diseases and young children for parents, teachers, and day care providers.

In Chapter 1, a brief history of communicable diseases and health care practices is presented. Public attitudes relative to health care and the historical foundations of public health are reviewed. Chapter 2 offers a short course in communicable disease, illness, and immunity. Terms are defined and concepts have been simplified for lay people. Chapter 3 offers an historical overview of early childhood education and a summary of contemporary practices related to the care and education of young children in groups. Chapter 4 delineates specific illnesses of concern in group settings. Chapter 5 offers recommendations for minimizing risks associated with the potential transmission of communicable diseases in group settings. In Chapter 6, legal issues likely to be associated with communicable diseases are described. Suggestions for minimizing liability exposure in group settings for young children are proposed for consideration. And finally, the Appendix offers a variety of resources for further information and guidance on communicable disease issues and young children. Professional organizations, informative publications, and reading material appropriate for use in health education activities with young children are listed and described.

J.M.T.

Acknowledgments

=== ====

We acknowledge, with many thanks, our professional families at the George Washington University, Sinai Hospital of Baltimore, and the University of New Mexico. We are particularly grateful for the support of Maxine Freund, Michael Castleberry, Teresa Rosegrant, Robert Ianacone, Phillip Goldstein, and Karen Engstrom. Their encouragement, continual good humor, and patience throughout this project was wonderful. We are also very grateful for the leadership provided by Michael Bender of the Kennedy Institute for Handicapped Children (Baltimore) in the preparation of this manuscript. Dr. Bender is an advisory editor for College-Hill Press and proposed development of a text related to communicable diseases and young children. We felt honored to be asked to pursue writing a project of this nature. Marie Linvill, the editor with College-Hill Press, offered encouragement and pragmatic recommendations from inception to completion of this manuscript. Suzanne Wagner, our lawyer and friend, reviewed the chapter on legal issues to assure its accuracy and inspired us by her warm, enthusiastic response. Ruth Luckasson, a scholar on legal issues related to persons with disabilities, also reviewed the legal issues chapter. She offered valuable information based on her preparation of a monograph for the American Bar Association, focusing on legal issues and acquired immunodeficiency syndrome (AIDS).

When the manuscript was nearly finished, our good friend Cheryl Trudil spent many tedious hours proofing our work and offering useful suggestions. We are certain the readability of the final document is due in great measure to Cheryl's fine assistance and her flair for words.

Others have bolstered us throughout the writing of this text. We consider each of these folks a good friend and colleague: Carol Ann Baglin, Dwight Baglin, Paula Beckman, Marjorie Shulbank, Ann Bailowitz,

Anita Roth, Sharon Goldstein, and Michael Hirsch. Our thanks and love to each of them.

And finally, we will be eternally indebted to our special supporters and cheerleaders, Rebecca Fewell, Deborah Deutsch Smith, and James Otto Smith. Their sage counsel has sustained us throughout the past decade, and their hospitality on our jaunts through the Southwest, Pacific Northwest, and now the Big Easy, has been delightful.

It is our hope that this text will enhance the efforts of parents and professionals to reduce illness among young children, staff members, and families. If you have any comments, criticisms, or suggestions, feel free to write to us in care of College-Hill Press. We would be delighted to have your feedback. Best wishes to each of you as you care for the most important resource in the world, our children.

J.M.T.
W.S.T.

Communicable Disease and
Young Children in Group Settings

CHAPTER 1

Historical Overview of Communicable Disease and Health Care

IMPORTANT TERMS

Infect   To infect is to enter, invade, or inhabit another
                          organism, causing infection or contamination.

Infectious   An infectious disease is one which is capable of
                          being transmitted by infection with or without
                          actual contact, also known as communicable.
                          The term also denotes a disease due to the action
                          of a microorganism (*Stedman's medical dictionary*,
                          1982).

HOW HAVE WE HISTORICALLY VIEWED COMMUNICABLE DISEASE?

PREHISTORIC SPECULATION AND FACTS

Perhaps the first disease was an infectious disease. It may have happened
that a young woman was scraping an animal hide in front of her nicely deco-
rated and tidy cave, when she gradually became aware of her skin becoming
hot, weakness in her arms and legs, and an uncontrollable shivering. When
her mate returned from the hunt, she might have grunted about feeling
poorly. He may have remained unconcerned for several days until he, too,
experienced the same combination of feelings. She probably died sometime
later after coughing and wasting away. He may have died from the same illness, but was more likely to have fallen prey to either an accident or a
wounded animal. Although this story is fictitious, it has been proven that
infectious diseases predate written history. Scientists have found evidence
of tuberculosis in the bones of humans who lived over 10,000 years ago.

BIBLICAL REFERENCES

One of our oldest written historical sources, the Bible, contains many references to infectious diseases. Some affected the course of history. For instance,
when the Egyptian pharaoh was subjected to a number of plagues, he was
compelled to release the Israelites. These plagues had many characteristics
of infectious diseases.

In the Old Testament there is a story about the Israelites and their peren-
nial enemy, the Philistines. After one of their frequent conflicts, the victori-
ous Philistines carried off the ark of the covenant only to suffer a plague of
epidemic proportions marked by the drainage of groin lumps (buboes). In

the same story there are references to "mice which mar the land." These are likely the first references to an epidemic of what we know as bubonic plague.

Leprosy is frequently mentioned in early historical and religious writings. It is probable that a person with any skin inflammation such as eczema or psoriasis was thought to have leprosy and isolated from the community. Lepers were considered unclean and were required to identify themselves as contaminated. They were our first social outcasts and bore the brunt of initial feeble attempts at public health and preventive medicine through isolation of diseased persons.

THE MIDDLE AGES

Although epidemics of disease occurred periodically in all European communities, they were usually short-lived and confined to relatively small geographic areas. As trade routes to the East were developed and religiously inspired crusades to the Holy Land were undertaken, the number of people afflicted increased. Leprosy continued to be recognized as a serious health threat in Europe centuries before the great plague epidemic of the fourteenth century. By the sixth century southern European governments were creating regulations which forbade free movement of lepers and mandated their isolation. In some areas lepers were declared legally dead or required to wear distinctive dress. Riesman (1935) states that some communities required lepers to wear a black coat with two white patches sewn on the breast and a tall hat with a white patch. During the thirteenth century only 12 diseases were thought to be contagious: leprosy, influenza, trachoma, ophthalmic gonorrhea, scabies, impetigo, typhus, anthrax, diphtheria, erysipelas, tuberculosis, and plague.

The bubonic plague, also known as the black death, began in the fourteenth century. It lasted 6 years and caused about 25 million deaths, approximately one fourth of the known European population. People were terrified and suspicious of one another. In some countries, those who frantically sought the cause of the plague accused Jews of trying to poison the world. In other countries, Christians were accused of the same crime. It became dangerous for any person to be seen touching a building with the fingers, for fear that a charge of poisoning would be lodged by the authorities. People accused one another of poisoning water through intentional contamination of wells. Some believed in astrological causes, and many believed the plague came from God as divine retribution for the continued sinfulness of the world (Riesman, 1935). It is interesting that the initial public response to acquired immunodeficiency syndrome (AIDS) some 600 years later was very much the same.

Methods for fighting the epidemic were interesting and varied. Doctors protected themselves by covering their bodies with long gowns, wearing gloves, and affixing sponges saturated with vinegar over their noses when ministering to plague victims. They advised light eating and avoidance of public gatherings. Rooms of sick people were aired and washed with vinegar or rose water. Physicians believed an acute illness ran its course in a maximum of 30 days. Plague victims and their families were customarily isolated, but due to the severity of this devastating illness, it became customary to extend the isolation period by an additional 10, or a total of 40 days. This number seemed especially appropriate because of its importance in biblical tradition. In the Italian language forty days is *quaranta giorni*, giving rise to the English word, "quarantine." Isolation and quarantine procedures became common practice and gradually led to the end of this widespread illness. Later, these measures became models of public health and hygiene practice and remain important tools of infection control. Although outbreaks continued to occur in subsequent years, lessons learned from this fourteenth-century epidemic minimized the consequences.

Between the fourteenth and twentieth centuries much scientific information about the nature of infectious disease was gathered. There were three important discoveries: the microscope by Leeuwenhoek, identification of bacteria and their relationship to illness by Pasteur, and Jenner's discovery of vaccines for disease prevention. As a result, concepts of public health and preventive medicine became important aspects of social and government concern. Many governmental programs were initiated, including: public sewage treatment, sanitary disposal systems, public water systems, water purity testing, immunization programs, food inspection, food distribution licensing, and occupational disease monitoring.

COMMUNICABLE DISEASE IN THE UNITED STATES

In preIndustrial United States, rural and small-town communities trusted their citizens to be capable of a wide range of skills and to be largely self-sufficient. This was certainly not an age of specialization. Each family supported the value of self-reliance. This tradition was born out of pioneer religious and political idealism. It is not surprising that early communities became accustomed to dealing with illness without the assistance of physicians (Starr, 1982). Doctors of that period were not held in high esteem. Few medical schools had standardized courses of study, and licencing of physicians was erratic. Doctors were self-appointed healers or itinerant entrepreneurs who hawked herbs and magic potions. These concoctions were usually based on folklore or family recipes. Occasionally some potions actually brought favorable results. Playing on the public's fears and igno-

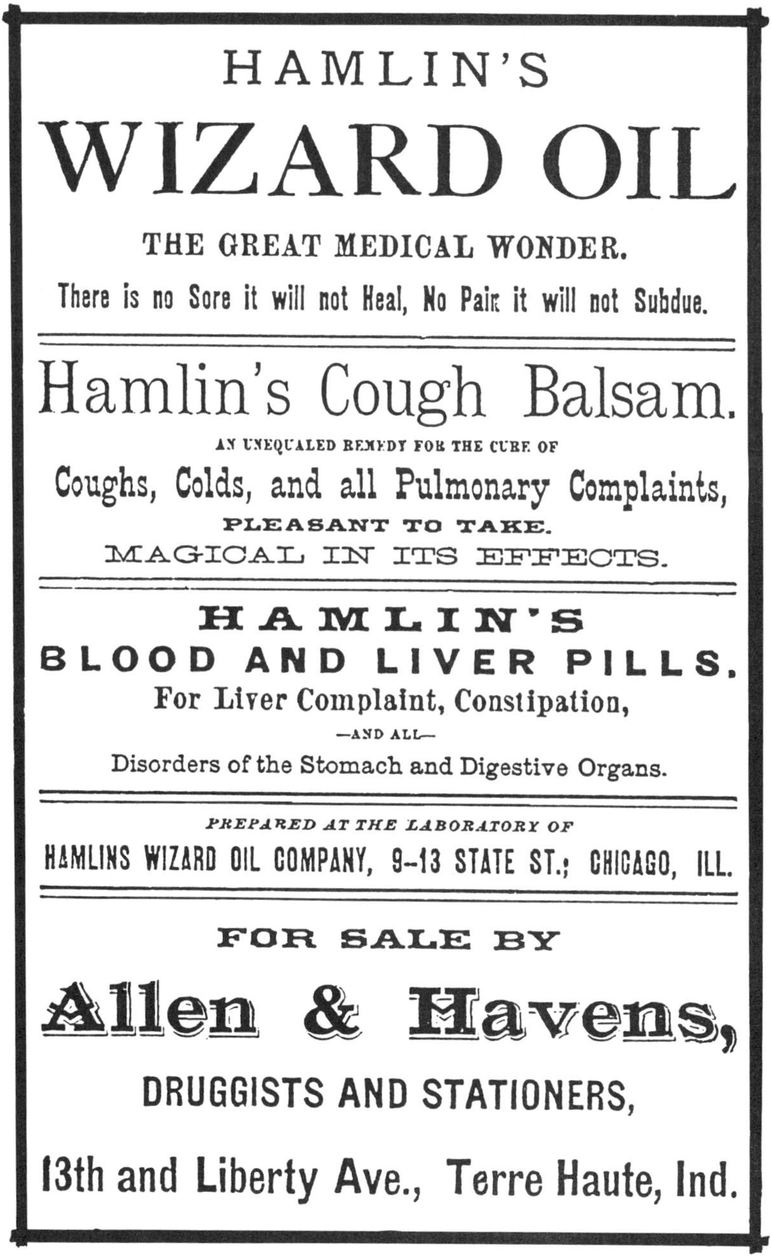

Figure 1-1. A nineteenth-century advertisement. (From Hechtlinger, A. [1970]. *The great patent medicine era.* New York: Grosset & Dunlap. Reprinted by permission.)

rance, vendors of "medicinals" marketed their products as guaranteed cures (Figure 1-1).

The majority of people lived on farms or in rural communities, without access to formally trained physicians. As a result, a large number of "healers" emerged and traveled from village to village. Drawing crowds by providing entertainment, these "medicine men" pitched their products and moved on before the efficacy of their medicines could be tested. Under the circumstances, it is not surprising that much of the burden of health care fell to women, where it remained until the early twentieth century.

Of course not all physicians were without credentials, but certainly the majority were. At the time of the American revolution it is estimated that there were 4,000 physicians, 400 of whom had formal medical training and perhaps another 200 with valid medical degrees (Starr, 1982). Prior to wide acceptance of women in professional occupations, formal systems of medical education in accredited medical schools were dominated by men. Physician organizations became powerful social, economic, and political groups.

THE TWENTIETH CENTURY

Contemporary society has been confronted by three major infectious diseases which have had profound social, political, and economic significance: influenza, poliomyelitis, and AIDS. Each of these is caused by a microorganism known as a virus.

INFLUENZA

This disease is a highly contagious respiratory illness which has afflicted humans for centuries. Although an early epidemic was reported by Hippocrates in 412 B.C., the worldwide epidemic, or pandemic, of 1918 and 1919 was particularly severe. It was called "Spanish influenza" and killed approximately 30 million people. The political and historical consequences were enormous. Approximately 80 percent of the U. S. Army deaths in World War I were due to influenza (Fields, 1985).

POLIOMYELITIS

Until recently, poliomyelitis was the best-known modern example of how an infectious disease spread through a community. The first sizeable outbreak in the United States occurred in Vermont in 1894, involving 132 cases. Recurrent and worsening outbreaks continued until 1955 when a polio vaccine was introduced. The effectiveness of the vaccine was demonstrated when reported cases declined from 38,000 to 570 cases per year (Fields, 1985).

ACQUIRED IMMUNODEFICIENCY SYNDROME

Acquired immunodeficiency syndrome (AIDS) was first reported in the United States in 1981. Considered a new disease, with an extraordinarily high fatality rate and no known cure or effective vaccine, AIDS has captured the attention of the public as no other disease in our generation. As of January 1988 there have been approximately 50,000 cases reported in the United States. It is estimated that an additional 2 million people have been infected with the virus, but have yet to manifest symptoms.

WHY DID GOVERNMENTS BECOME INVOLVED IN HEALTH ISSUES?

PUBLIC HEALTH

Public health programs began when concerned citizens noticed that epidemics occurred more frequently in crowded, impoverished areas. Accumulation of garbage or sewage assured the arrival of insects, rodents, and eventually disease. It seemed reasonable to assume that sanitation would control disease. Citizens insisted on governmental involvement. Waste disposal and control became prime government concerns. When public sanitation programs were instituted, contagious disease lessened.

Further attempts to organize a nationwide system of public health were resisted by medicine men and trained physicians who perceived health care as the exclusive dominion of the private practitioner. For several years doctors fought public treatment of patients, reporting of tuberculosis and venereal disease, and attempts to coordinate preventive and curative medical services (Starr, 1982). Nevertheless, states and local communities eventually developed health departments.

Louisiana established the first state board of health in 1855. Other states and some cities made similar attempts, but few were successful initially. Finally, by the end of the nineteenth century, New York City established the first successful public health department in the face of both active and passive opposition by many physicians. In fact, the New York program influenced national public health practices. New York City's health department introduced laboratory diagnosis of communicable disease, produced and distributed vaccines and sera, registered cases of tuberculosis and venereal diseases, provided health education, and established school health programs. Physicians gradually accepted public health programs. Physicians and public health officials began to work toward common goals (Starr, 1982).

SCHOOL HEALTH SERVICES

Public health efforts on behalf of schoolchildren were directed at improving building ventilation and heating. A proper learning environment was the main concern. Initially, smallpox vaccination was the only medical service occasionally provided through school systems. As public health services expanded, school health programs focused on medical problems, including communicable diseases. In 1894, Boston became the first city to employ school inspectors to identify and send home ill children. A few years later, New York City appointed school inspectors to identify children with infectious diseases. School health programs gradually included vision and hearing testing. Eventually, school health officials screened students for other problems which might interfere with learning. Unfortunately inspectors had minimal contact with parents, and families often had little money, so health problems that were discovered in educational settings were often not treated. Officials employed health care workers in schools in an attempt to solve this problem, leading to routine use of school nurses in New York City in 1902 (Starr, 1982).

HOW IS GOVERNMENT CURRENTLY INVOLVED IN HEALTH ISSUES?

GOVERNMENTAL POLICY AND PUBLIC HEALTH

The response of nations to public health issues is extremely varied, relating to a variety of factors including culture, tradition, philosophy, economics, and resources. In the Constitution of the United States, there is no mention of governmental responsibility for public health. *Most policies having to do with communicable disease are implemented by states on advice and authority of state health agencies.* One federally sponsored agency in the United States is the Centers for Disease Control (CDC) in Atlanta, Georgia. The CDC monitors health through the accumulation and interpretation of epidemiologic data, conducts research, and makes recommendations for disease control. This agency is a valuable source of current information about past and present infectious disease problems.

SUMMARY

For most of human history the nature of infectious disease has been a mystery and a source of unrelenting fear. Illness was perceived as a form of divine justice. Sick people were avoided or isolated lest they contaminate others.

With the discovery that germs cause infectious disease, a portion of the mystery was solved. Scientists developed tests, discovered cures, and provided information that was useful in preventing the spread of disease. This information has become the basis for many policies in federal, state, and health agencies, and has resulted in a number of programs which affect children, caretakers, and educators. There are now minimum standards and requirements relating to public health issues throughout the United States and trust territories.

SUGGESTED READING

Starr, P. (1982). *The social transformation of American medicine.* New York: Basic Books.

CHAPTER 2

Microbiology and Immunology Made Easy

IMPORTANT TERMS

Antigen An antigen is that portion of the biological structure of a microorganism which identifies it as being foreign to the host.

Antibody An antibody is a substance produced by certain white blood cells (lymphocytes) in response to contact with an antigen; also called *immunoglobulin*.

Carrier A carrier is an individual who is infected by an organism but is not "sick," and therefore has no symptoms or signs of illness.

Contact A contact is a person known to have been in close contact with, *and* presumably exposed to an infected person or object(s) handled by an infected person.

Incubation period Incubation period is the time interval from the entrance of an organism into a host until sickness is apparent.

Microbiology Microbiology is a branch of biology dealing with microscopic life forms.

Sign Medically, a sign is an *objective* manifestation of disease, such as a fever or rash.

Symptom A symptom is a *subjective* complaint of a person afflicted with a disease, such as pain or weakness.

Virulence Virulence is the power of a microorganism to cause a disease in a given host.

WHAT ARE THE ABCs OF COMMUNICABLE DISEASE?

In order to understand the consequences of infectious disease in group settings for young children, it is helpful to be familiar with *microbiology*. Microbiology is the study of microscopic living things called microorganisms, or

Table 2-1. THE STUDY OF MICROBIOLOGY

Subdivision	*Organism*
Bacteriology	Bacteria
Virology	Viruses
Mycology	Fungi
Protozoology	Protozoa
Parasitology	Parasites

germs (Table 2-1). There are five classifications of microorganisms: bacteria, viruses, fungi, protozoa, and parasites. Any of these organisms can cause disease. In children, bacteria and viruses are the most common causes of serious communicable diseases.

We are constantly surrounded by huge numbers of microorganisms. In a silent struggle, potentially hazardous infectious organisms wage a constant battle with the human body for supremacy (Wehrle and Franklin, 1981). To survive, microorganisms need a *host*. The host provides basic nutrients for growth and reproduction. Microorganisms, therefore, are essentially parasites and must find a host for survival. Once a host has been found, microorganisms seem to be biologically programmed for survival. They use the host's tissues for food and reproduce themselves to assure continuity of the species. It is disadvantageous to the organism to cause death or destruction of its host, for then, its own survival would be limited.

THE DISEASE PROCESS

With few exceptions the development of a communicable disease follows a consistent pattern. First, an organism enters the body. Entrance can be gained through one of several routes: skin, nose, throat, lungs, intestines, genitalia, or urinary system. Next a favorable site is located to launch the initial attack. It is still unknown why microorganisms invade some cells and not others, but once located they multiply, disrupting the structure and function of host cells. This disruption is called a *primary* lesion. From the primary lesion organisms may spread to surrounding cells or tissues, or gain access to the circulatory system. Once in the circulatory system, organisms can travel rapidly to distant areas of the body, producing *secondary* lesions.

The end of an illness is usually marked by elimination of organisms and subsequent disappearance of symptoms and signs. However, some viruses or bacteria persist within the body for months or years producing little or no

Figure 2-1. Bacterial growth curve.

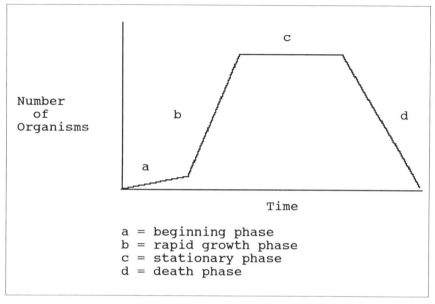

```
Number
  of
Organisms
```
Time

a = beginning phase
b = rapid growth phase
c = stationary phase
d = death phase

disease. This condition is called the *carrier* state and can be caused by a number of factors, including the microorganism's strength or *virulence*, impairent of normal defense mechanisms which fight against disease, and the ability of some viruses to escape detection by normal defense mechanisms. These persistent viruses may reactivate at a later time producing acute disease again, or may result in a chronic carrier state.

BACTERIA

Microorganisms, like humans, need certain conditions for successful growth, reproduction, and continued life. Scientists have discovered that bacteria have a life cycle very similar to that seen in larger human populations (Figure 2-1). In the *beginning phase*, the organism is adjusting to the environment. During the *rapid growth phase* new cell material is produced and the population increases. At a certain point the number of new organisms produced is exactly equal to the number that die. This balanced state is called the *stationary phase*. Finally, when nutrients are exhausted and there is a large amount of "sewage," organisms die faster than they reproduce. These events mark the *death phase*.

Table 2-2. LOCATION AND IDENTITY OF NORMAL HUMAN FLORA

Site	Organism
Mouth	Staphylococci
	Streptococci
	Bacilli
	Candida (yeasts)
Nose and throat	Staphylococci
	Streptococci
	Neisseria
	Lactobacilli
	Bacteroides
	Haemophilus
Intestine	Staphylococci
	Streptococci
	Escherichia coli
	Proteus
	Lactobacilli
	Bacteroides
	Enterococcus
	Candida (yeasts)

NORMAL BACTERIA

The skin, upper respiratory system (mouth, nose, and throat), and intestinal system are populated by a variety of "friendly" bacteria. Under normal circumstances they do not cause disease, but actually assist in preventing invasion by harmful organisms. These organisms are called *normal flora*. Table 2-2 contains a list of normal flora and their usual locations. Characteristics of normal flora in an individual are greatly influenced by diet, climate, social customs, race, and other factors. Disease is usually produced by a new, harmful organism. However, when the normal defense mechanisms of the body are faulty, even normal flora can produce disease.

Skin

Skin is the largest organ of the human body. Although normally populated by many organisms, the amount and kind are dependent on proximity to body openings. For instance, facial skin is populated by a large number of bacteria similar to those in the mouth, nose, and throat. Skin of the genital area is populated by organisms similar to those in the intestines.

Mouth

Prior to birth, a newborn has few bacteria in the mouth. During the birth process, normal flora from the mother's vagina gain access to the infant's mouth. These are usually harmless bacteria and are gradually replaced by others. It is normal for the mouth to be inhabited by a large number and variety of bacteria.

Nose and Throat

Bacteria from the air are filtered by the nose and throat and become lodged in mucus-producing linings. They are predominantly streptococci and are considered part of the normal flora.

Intestines

Most organisms entering the digestive system are killed by stomach acids. Therefore, the stomach and the first part of the small intestine are typically sterile. However, further down the intestinal tract there is a more favorable environment for bacterial growth. Large numbers of normal flora, predominately, *Escherichia* (E. coli), live in the large intestine.

DISEASE-CAUSING BACTERIA

Bacteria which are able to produce disease are called *pathogenic*. It is important to realize that *normal flora can become pathogenic when the balance between the body's defense mechanisms and its normal flora is interrupted*.

VIRUSES

Viruses are the smallest microorganisms. They reproduce and infect people in entirely different ways than bacteria. After a cell is invaded, bacteria reproduce themselves by a simple process of growth and repeated division. When nutrients stored in the cell are exhausted by increasing numbers of bacteria, cell death occurs. The bacteria then find new cells to support growth. Viruses do not reproduce by simple division. They have an astounding ability to program the metabolic activities of host cells to produce identical copies of themselves. Eventually, a cell becomes overwhelmed and dies. Viruses then search for another cell and the cycle is repeated. Table 2-3 lists the classification of some infectious viruses and examples of illnesses they cause.

Since viruses do not behave like bacteria, growth curves, temperature, tissue acidity, and nutrient requirements may not be comparable or even rele-

Table 2-3. CLASSIFICATION OF VIRUSES AND SOME VIRAL DISEASES

Class	*Disease Example*
Adenoviruses	Colds
Arboviruses	Yellow fever
Arenaviruses	Lassa fever
Coronaviruses	Colds
Cytomegalovirus (CMV)	CMV disease
Enteroviruses	Hepatitis
	Poliomyelitis
	Meningitis
Epstein-Barr virus	Infectious mononucleosis
Rotaviruses	Gastroenteritis
Herpes simplex virus	Oral or genital infection
Influenza viruses	Respiratory infection
Rabies virus	Rabies
Respiratory syncytial virus	Respiratory infections
Rhinoviruses	Respiratory infections
Rubella virus	German measles
Varicella-zoster virus	Chickenpox
Retroviruses	Acquired immunodeficiency syndrome (AIDS)

vant. Each cell provides characteristics necessary for survival of a virus. Scientists have identified few viruses which are considered normal inhabitants of the human body.

HOW ARE COMMUNICABLE DISEASES TRANSMITTED?

The ways in which bacteria and viruses are passed from one person to another are identical. In health care sciences these are known as "routes of transmission." Bacterial infections are frequently eliminated through the use of antibiotics. There are no known cures for most viral infections. Since viruses seem to cause problems more frequently than bacteria, discussion of transmission will focus on viral diseases.

RESPIRATORY

Spread of viral illness occurs most commonly via the respiratory system. Coughing, sneezing, and breathing fill the air with microscopic water droplets which transport viruses from one host to another. The intensity of a cough or sneeze and the amount of mucus discharged from mouth and nose affect the likelihood of viral transmission. Viruses can also enter the respiratory system by direct contact. Kissing or mouthing contaminated objects would be considered direct contact. Researchers have found that concentrations of certain respiratory viruses are highest on fingers and hands; therefore *frequent hand washing has been recommended for control of the common cold* (Evans, 1982).

GASTROINTESTINAL

If good hand-washing techniques are not used after toileting, it is possible for microorganisms which are present in body wastes to be deposited on objects. These might be mouthed by another person. This is called the *oral-fecal* route of transmission. Among young children the oral-fecal route of viral transmission is fairly common because they are novice hand washers and tend to lack the maturity to use good judgment regarding hygiene. Food handlers who do not wash thoroughly after toileting can cause microorganisms to be transferred to food, which may be eaten by others. Transmission by the oral-fecal route is the second most frequent way viruses are spread.

Viruses pass from mouth to stomach and along the intestinal tract until they find susceptible cells. At this point viruses may cause local tissue injury producing symptoms such as cramping or diarrhea. Certain viruses pass through intestinal cells without injuring them, into the bloodstream where they can travel to distant areas in the body until an appropriate site is found. For instance, the hepatitis virus travels to the liver where it sets up residence, causing injury to cells. This virus is shed from the liver to the intestinal tract and can infect others via the oral-fecal route of transmission. Since fecal contamination of hands, food, water, toys, or other articles may cause hepatitis, *thorough hand washing after toileting or handling of contaminated items is extremely important*. Viruses that are spread through this route are easier to control environmentally than viruses transmitted through the respiratory route (Evans, 1982).

SKIN

Penetration of intact skin is an unlikely method of viral transmission. Although relatively uncommon, animal bites can transmit rabies, mosquito bites can cause yellow fever, and use of nonsterile needles for injections or transfusion with infected blood can cause some kinds of hepatitis or spread the human immunodeficiency virus (HIV), the cause of acquired immunodeficiency syndrome (AIDS). Typically, infection through skin penetration is an issue in programs for children only when hepatitis B carriers or HIV carriers exhibit problem behaviors, like biting or scratching.

When skin openings occur due to cuts, abrasions, or conditions like eczema, viruses can enter the body. To minimize risks of contracting communicable disease through the skin, cuts, lesions, scratches, and other openings should be covered when possible. Generally, clothing provides an adequate barrier against microorganisms, but rubber gloves, Band-Aids, or other dressings may be used. For specific advice, consult appropriate health care providers.

In addition to infection by skin penetration, certain viruses have a tendency to attack specific tissue, including skin tissue. For example, the virus that causes chickenpox tends to attack the skin. The result is small, fluid-filled blisters, characteristic of chickenpox. Chickenpox lesions contain large numbers of live viruses. As a result, lesions on the skin become a potential source of infection to others.

GENITAL

As a baby passes through the birth canal, the genital area can be a source of infection for infants. Viruses causing herpes simplex, cytomegaloinclusion disease, and AIDS have all been isolated from genital tract secretions. Newborns have less immunity than adults and are especially susceptible to infection, even during the birth process. Often, infections acquired before or during birth can be manifested by serious developmental problems, mental retardation, seizure disorders, or chronic, multiple skin lesions.

INTRAUTERINE OR TRANSPLACENTAL

As previously suggested, an infant can acquire an infection during passage through the birth canal. Furthermore, an unborn baby can become infected by microorganisms in the mother's bloodstream that pass across the placental barrier to the unborn baby's bloodstream. This is known as transplacental (across the placenta) transmission of infection which causes intrauterine (inside the uterus) infection. Intrauterine infections tend to be serious and may affect an infant's developmental outcome. Viruses which can produce infections transplacentally include herpesvirus, cytomegalovirus (CMV), hepatitis B, rubella (German measles), varicella (chickenpox), and HIV. CMV and rubella are probably the most common congenital viral infections (Evans, 1982).

Table 2-4. TRANSMISSION OF VIRAL DISEASES

Exit	Route of Transmission	Entry	Example
Respiratory	Salivary	Respiratory	Influenza
	Aerosol	Mouth	Herpes
Intestinal	Stool-hand	Mouth	Hepatitis A
	Stool-food	Mouth	Hepatitis A
Skin	Skin to skin	Abraded skin	Herpes, warts
Blood	Needles	Skin	Hepatitis B, acquired immunodeficiency syndrome (AIDS)
Urine	Uncertain	Uncertain	Cytomegalic inclusion disease
Genital	Genital	Genital secretions	Herpes, AIDS
Placental	Directly to fetus	Blood	Cytomegalic inclusion disease, AIDS, rubella

Adapted from Evans, A. S. (1982). *Viral infections in humans* (p. 10). New York: Plenum.

URINARY

It is currently believed that urinary transmission of microorganisms is of minor importance because the urinary tract is generally sterile and inhospitable. Transmission of CMV is an exception. CMV is excreted in urine.

In group settings of young children, toileting accidents and diaper changing can be sources of viral transmission through contact with urine. Again, the importance of good hand-washing routines must be emphasized.

Transmission of some viral diseases is demonstrated in Table 2-4. This summary is by no means complete. A fuller explanation is offered by Evans (1982).

WHAT ARE THE ABCs OF RESISTANCE?

NATURAL DEFENSE MECHANISMS

We are constantly surrounded by billions of microorganisms. The frequency, severity, and duration of any infectious process is related to the efficiency of a very complex resistance system which is simplified in Figure 2-2. *An infectious illness will occur only when this intricate system is overwhelmed.*

Given the number and variety of disease-producing bacteria and viruses surrounding humans, it seems fortunate that anyone survives childhood. In fact, most people die from degenerative processes, not infections. As a result

Figure 2-2. The struggle for health.

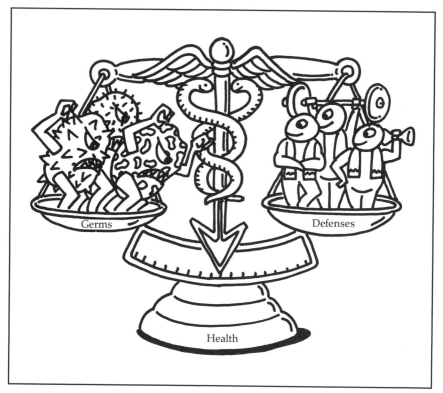

of public health programs, immunizations, diagnostic testing, and discovery of antibiotics, risks of infectious disease have been reduced tremendously in this century. Also, the human body has a vast array of protective mechanisms which function quite well under normal circumstances. These protective mechanisms are collectively known as the *immune system* and can be divided into *physical factors*, *nonspecific factors*, and *specific factors*.

PHYSICAL FACTORS

Unbroken skin

This is the initial barrier to infection. With very few exceptions organisms cannot pass through the skin into underlying tissues. If the skin is injured, even by a small puncture, organisms can enter the body and cause an infection. Neglect of skin injuries can allow even more organisms to enter the body.

Respiratory Tract

The entire respiratory tract is lined by cells which produce mucous secretions. Dust, microorganisms, and other particles which can cause infection are trapped by the secretions. Cells in the respiratory tract also have minute hairlike structures called *cilia* which continually move trapped particles toward the nose and throat where they are expelled by coughing or sneezing.

Gastrointestinal system

Normal stomach secretions contain gastric acid which kills many organisms. Surviving microorganisms are usually destroyed by secretions in the upper portion of the small intestine.

Genitourinary system

Protection against invasion by microorganisms via genitourinary openings is provided by a thick layer of cells lining these structures. Further, secretions and acidity of the area provide an inhospitable environment for the growth of microorganisms.

NONSPECIFIC IMMUNITY FACTORS

Certain white blood cells monitor purity of the bloodstream and other body tissues. They can recognize microorganisms as foreign invaders and physically destroy them. If the number or virulence of invading organisms overwhelms this first line of defense, a second mechanism begins to function. The body attempts to keep infection localized to a small area by using a system of filters. This is called the *lymphatic system* and is composed of small lymphatic vessels and lymph nodes. The most frequently recognized lymph nodes are located in the neck near the lower jawbone. These can become enlarged, tender, or painful when a person has an infection, for example, a sore throat. These lymph nodes are often referred to as "swollen glands." If the second line of defense, the lymphatic system, fails and microorganisms escape to other parts of the body, the result is a *fever*. At this point other defenses begin to function.

SPECIFIC IMMUNITY FACTORS

In addition to general recognition of foreign invaders, certain white blood cells called *lymphocytes* have the ability to recognize *antigens*, the chemical and biological structures of invading microorganisms. Each microorganism has

Figure 2-3. Immune system function.

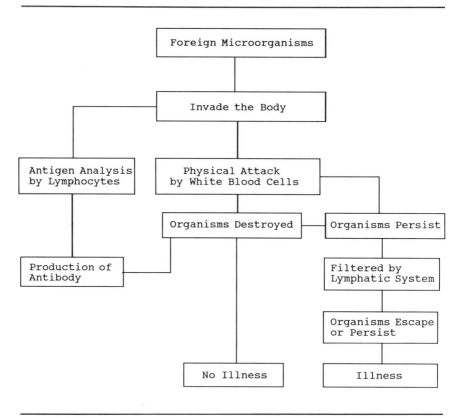

its own specific and unique *antigenic structure*. Lymphocytes can use information gained by analyzing the antigen to produce a specific and unique "poison," called *antibody*, or immunoglobulin (Ig). This antibody circulates in the bloodstream and is distributed to all infected tissues. Antibodies either destroy or neutralize invading microorganisms. Unfortunately, antigen recognition and antibody production is not a rapid process, but once the antibody is produced it usually lasts for several months or years. When antibodies persist, a state of *immunity* is said to exist. Figure 2-3 diagrams this complex system.

Initially all antibody was thought to have similar characteristics, but in recent times scientists have found distinct groups which are identified by the following abbreviations:

IgM

IgM is the first antibody to appear on exposure to any antigen. IgM does not persist for long periods of time and is gradually replaced by other antibodies. IgM manufactured by the mother does not cross the placenta. Finding high levels of IgM in a newborn indicates the presence of an infection acquired before birth, like rubella or CMV.

IgG

IgG is an important antibody. In the face of an infection, IgG accumulates slowly and persists for long periods of time. IgG passes through the placenta of a pregnant woman and provides some protection for newborns. Because of the vigor of its response to microorganisms and certain toxins, IgG can be used to prevent or lessen the effects of certain diseases, like measles or hepatitis A.

Other Antibodies

There are additional groups of antibodies. They will not be addressed in this text as they are not believed to be significant to communicable disease and young children in group settings.

Cellular Immunity Functions

Other lymphocytes provide protective functions aside from antibody production. These complex activities are grouped together as cellular immunity functions. Medical researchers are studying these intensely in an effort to combat many diseases, including AIDS and cancer.

ACQUIRED DEFENSE MECHANISMS

Immunization

In some ways, smallpox was more devastating than the plague. Approximately 80 percent of the world population was infected with smallpox and 25 percent of those infected either died or were severely disfigured. Smallpox did not distinguish between rich or poor people as it was contracted in equal numbers by both (Gross and Levine, 1987).

Late in the eighteenth century, Edward Jenner described a technique of injecting a small amount of cowpox virus into the skin of the arm, a process

Table 2-5. IMMUNIZATION SCHEDULE

Recommended Age	Vaccine(s)
2 months	1st DPT, 1st OP
4 months	2nd DPT, 2nd OP
6 months	3rd DPT
15 months	4th DPT, MMR, 3rd OP
24 months	HbV (for those at increased risk, e.g., child care students)
4¢6 years	5th DPT, 4th OP
14¢16 years	Td (repeated every 10 years)

DPT = diphtheria, pertussis, tetanus vaccine; OP = oral polio vaccine; MMR = measles, mumps, rubella vaccine; HbV = *Haemophilus* B vaccine; Td = tetanus and diphtheria toxoid vaccine.

called vaccination. He discovered that persons vaccinated with cowpox virus (which does not cause disease in humans) became immune to smallpox. Jenner's process led to the discovery of a more inclusive process called immunization. Immunity to other diseases was provided by administering a variety of biological agents.

The concept of immunization is directly related to antigen identification and antibody production. When a person is infected with a microorganism, becomes ill, produces antibody, and recovers, the antibody often persists for a long time. This naturally acquired *immunity* is the result of antibody persistence. Scientists have been able to find ways to produce immunity without causing illness by altering microorganisms. If a susceptible person is given a dose of altered organisms, antibody will be produced and immunity will result. This is called *active immunity*. Another process, called *passive immunity*, involves extracting antibody from the blood of a large number of previously infected people or animals, purifying it, and then injecting it into susceptible persons. Active immunity is slow in onset, but long-lasting. Passive immunity is rapid in onset, but temporary. The appropriate immunization depends on the nature of the disease, characteristics of exposure, and infectious disease history of each individual.

Current immunization policy is available from many sources including the American Academy of Pediatrics (AAP), local health agencies, local physicians, hospitals, and the Centers for Disease Control (CDC). Based on AAP and CDC guidelines, a recommended schedule for active immunization of normal infants and children is listed in Table 2-5. There are other recommended immunization schedules (available from the same sources) for children who were not immunized at the recommended time, for unimmunized persons over the age of 7 years, and for children with HIV infection.

SUMMARY

The study of infectious disease is the study of microorganisms and how they are classified, gain access to susceptible persons, and cause disease. Microorganisms are everywhere, and are present in large numbers on every body surface that is exposed to the environment. Most microorganisms are harmless in normal situations. Fortunately, those which are especially virulent are uncommon.

The study of infectious disease includes the study of *immunology*. Once an organism gains a foothold in a susceptible person, defense mechanisms are triggered to inactivate invaders. White blood cells in general, and especially lymphocytes, direct the inactivation or destruction of offending organisms. Using information gained from microbiology and immunology, scientists have developed agents which can prevent or lessen the severity of a large number of diseases. This process is called *immunization*.

SUGGESTED READING

Braunwald, E., Isselbacher, K. J., Petersdorf, R. G., Wilson, J. D., Martin, J. B., and Fauci, A. S. (Eds.). (1987). *Harrison's principles of internal medicine* (11th ed.). New York: McGraw-Hill.

Dubay, E. C., and Grubb, R. D. (1978). *Infection prevention and control* (2nd ed.). St. Louis, MO: C. V. Mosby.

Fields, B. N. (Ed.). (1985). *Virology.* New York: Raven Press.

Jaroff, L. (1988, May 23). The battle inside your body. *Time,* pp. 56–64.

Remington, J. S., and Klein, J. O. (Eds.). (1983). *Infectious diseases of the fetus and newborn infant.* Philadelphia, PA: W. B. Saunders.

CHAPTER 3

*Young Children and
Group Settings*

IMPORTANT TERMS

Child care   Child care is the placement of children in out- of-home settings while parents or guardians work, attend school, or are involved in other activities.

Early childhood programs   Early childhood programs are educational child care arrangements for young children under the age of 8 years.

WHY HAVE GROUP SETTINGS FOR YOUNG CHILDREN?

CHILD CARE

Child care has become increasingly necessary. In the last few decades, there have been dramatic increases in the number of children cared for by someone other than a parent. By the year 1990, it is anticipated that approximately 11 million children under the age of 6 years will be enrolled in child care while parents work or attend school. Most child care arrangements involve group settings for young children (Children's Defense Fund, 1986).

Most parents need time away from their children. Ilg and Ames (1955) suggest that preschools can be useful for parents. Early childhood programs offer a "time of relief from the constant twenty-four-hour care of a preschooler...[and] an opportunity to talk over daily problems...with trained and sympathetic teachers" (p. 257). As described in a publication of the Yale Bush Center in Child Development and Social Policy (Payne, 1983), "Parenting is a tough job. ... Parents are also people with their own needs" (p.3). Time away from children is one of those needs. Babysitters, relatives, day care providers, and other caretakers offer respite opportunities for parents of young children.

EARLY EDUCATION

John Amos Comenius (1592–1670), a Moravian minister from Czechoslovakia, is thought to have been the first advocate of universal education in a child's formative years. Comenius believed young minds should be prepared to receive information in order to avoid moral corruption. Other philosophers and educators have echoed Comenius's sentiments and refined his concepts. A variety of early childhood education approaches have emerged, including developmental, theoretical, behavioral, Piagetian, Montessori, and the cognitively oriented. Central to each theoretical approach is the importance of group activities. Group learning and interaction are believed to foster social, emotional, and intellectual development (Morrison 1988). Children spend time with others for storytelling, snacks, playground activities, field trips, and many other learning experiences.

PREVENTION OF DEVELOPMENTAL DELAYS

Some children are at risk for experiencing delays in development. Children from high-risk groups include children born to mentally retarded, psychiatrically disordered, abusive, or teenage parents. Many of these children are eligible for compensatory preschool programs designed to minimize effects of parental and environmental risk factors (Fraas, 1986).

Head Start has been the most widely publicized compensatory preschool effort in the United States. Typically, children enroll in Head Start programs after age 3 years. Some centers accept younger children.

SPECIAL PROGRAMS FOR CHILDREN WITH IDENTIFIED DEVELOPMENTAL DELAYS

In special programs for young children, developmental assessments are conducted to determine a child's status with respect to social, emotional, fine motor, gross motor, communication, self-help, cognitive, and sensory development. If testing indicates a lag in one or more areas of a child's development, enrollment in a special infant or preschool program can be beneficial. Social development activities are usually stressed, and when possible, developmentally delayed children and nonhandicapped peers spend time together. This is believed to promote normalization of the child's early experiences (Bricker, 1986; Guralnick, 1978).

RECREATION AND RELIGION

Recreation

Franchised recreational programs designed for young children have gained popularity in the past decade. Play groups, swim classes, gymnastics, organized sports, and exercise classes for children or parent-child dyads are increasingly available.

Religion

Children may participate in religious training from an early age. Religious classes, services, and meetings can be a regular part of a child's week. Children of devout families can spend significant amounts of time in group activities sponsored by religious organizations.

WHY ARE COMMUNICABLE DISEASES A PROBLEM IN GROUP SETTINGS FOR YOUNG CHILDREN?

PHYSICAL FACTORS

The most common reason for contracting any illness is contact with others. Therefore, as children spend time with adults or other children, especially nonfamily members, the potential for infectious disease transmission increases.

Very young children are more susceptible to illness than older children. The natural immunity an infant acquires from its maternal antibodies lasts only a few weeks or months. A baby is therefore more vulnerable to infection until additional protective antibodies are acquired (Klein, 1986).

The size and position of eustachian tubes in young children increases the likelihood that a common cold will lead to an ear infection (otitis media). Ear infections tend to occur with greatest frequency in children who are between 10 and 18 months of age. By age 3 years, two thirds of all children have had at least one ear infection and one third of all children have had three or more. As a child reaches school age, the eustachian tube has lengthened, narrowed, and protects the middle ear from infection to a greater degree. By first grade, ear infections are relatively uncommon (Klein, 1986).

Additionally, there are several illnesses that occur primarily in early childhood. For example, the incidence of meningitis is highest during the first 3 years of life (Klein, 1986).

COMMUNICATION

Preverbal children are unable to communicate specific health complaints to parents and caretakers. Language skills are not developed enough to describe aches and pains. Rashes, cuts, sores, and flushed skin can be observed; however, other ailments can only be surmised. For example, a young child's crying or whining may be a sign of a stomachache, headache, or sore joints. Parents, caretakers, and health care providers must play detective to ascertain the exact cause of the malady. Therefore, some symptoms associated with communicable diseases may go undetected when a child is contagious.

SOCIAL BEHAVIORS

Common social behaviors of young children can increase the likelihood of spreading infectious diseases. Very young children drool and routinely explore objects by mouthing. Saliva deposited on toys can contain viral or bacterial particles. If infected toys are shared, germs may be transferred from one child to another.

Klein (1986) describes another behavior which undoubtedly contributes to the transmission of communicable disease. Children between the ages of 1 and 5 years were found to put "a hand or object in their mouth every three minutes" (p. 522).

Normally developing toddlers and preschoolers eventually outgrow drooling and mouthing. New behaviors emerge, among them greater control over hand and mouth movements. Children are now able to spit, scratch, bite, share food, or "play doctor." These can lead to an exchange of body fluids, for example, blood or mucus. Nevertheless, it is generally agreed that the benefits of social contacts are thought to outweigh the infection risks associated with group settings (Centers for Disease Control, 1985).

SELF-HELP BEHAVIORS

Children lacking bowel or bladder control must have diapers changed regularly. Since feces and urine of sick children contain infectious germs, toileting accidents or poor hygiene can contribute to the spread of illness. Youngsters with newly acquired toilet skills may lack thoroughness in their clean-up attempts. Soiled clothing may be handled improperly, attempts at "wiping" may be futile, or hands may not be washed adequately. Further, the "aim" of boys who are novice toilet users may prove imperfect.

Eating habits can also contribute to the spread of infection. Young children sneeze on snacks, share food after taking bites, or eat food which has fallen on the floor. The most vigilant caretaker would find it difficult to foresee and prevent every unsanitary event.

Oozing sores or lesions containing infectious particles, such as those caused by herpes simplex viruses, should be covered to minimize potential transmission of viral particles. Young children may not understand the importance of keeping a lesion covered and remove Band-Aids or neglect to inform caretakers if a Band-Aid is accidentally dislodged.

ECONOMIC PRESSURE

Parents often feel pressured to leave their children with a caretaker even if the child is ill. Children less than 3 years of age tend to contract 7 to 9 respiratory illnesses per year (Klein, 1986). Each bout lasts approximately 6 days. Working parents are often faced with limited leave policies which make it difficult to stay home with a sick child. Parents may lose income or their job if they take excessive time from work to care for an ill child. "Illness in children is a leading cause of industrial absenteeism among working parents" (p. 523). Although day care for ill children has become available in some areas, it is limited and tends to be prohibitively expensive. Thus, parents may feel forced to send contagious children to day care centers.

TRANSPORTATION

Car pools or vans are often used to transport children to babysitters, preschools, and child care centers. Although researchers have yet to focus on this issue, Klein (1986) suggests that infection during transport could account for a significant number of illnesses.

Imagine a station wagon with windows shut in midwinter with eight to ten toddlers shouting, laughing, sneezing, coughing, and wrestling for 30 minutes twice a day. A communicable infection in one child is likely to be shared with all children and adults in the vehicle. (p. 523)

PHYSICAL FACILITIES

A number of factors related to physical facilities may account for communicable disease transmission. Contributing factors can include space allotment per child (e.g., during nap time), ventilation, cleanliness of food preparation and eating areas, availability of sinks with running water, separation of food preparation or eating areas from diaper-changing areas, and susceptibility of surfaces to habitation by microorganisms.

SUMMARY

Currently, millions of young children spend time in group settings outside the home. Day care, special infant programs, preschools, religious organizations, and recreational facilities provide opportunities for children to interact with nonfamily members. Most group settings are not sterile and contain organisms capable of causing infection. Contamination cannot be avoided. Contact with other humans inevitably involves a degree of risk with respect to illness. It is crucial that parents, teachers, and other caretakers of young children familiarize themselves with techniques for minimizing transmission of communicable diseases.

SUGGESTED READING

Bricker, D. D. (1986). *Early education of at-risk and handicapped infants, toddlers, and preschool children*. Glenview, IL: Scott, Foresman.

Brown, J. F. (Ed.). (1984). *Administering programs for young children*. Washington, DC: National Association for the Education of Young Children.

Decker, C. A., and Decker, J. R. (1984). *Planning and administering early childhood programs* (3rd ed.). Columbus, OH: Charles E. Merrill.

Guralnick, M. J., and Bennett, F. J. (1987). *The effectiveness of early intervention for at-risk and handicapped children*. New York: Academic Press.

Morrison, G. S. (1988). *Early childhood education today* (4th ed.). Columbus, OH: Charles E. Merrill.

CHAPTER 4

Communicable Diseases and Group Settings for Young Children

IMPORTANT TERMS

Reportable disease   A reportable disease is one which, according to state or local statute or regulation, must be reported to public health officials because of the possibility of spread within a community.

Shedding   Shedding is continued excretion of infectious microorganisms, often persisting for long periods of time even after the illness has subsided.

Immunoglobulin   Immunoglobulin is the scientific name for antibody.

Immune globulin   Immune globulin is the scientific name for an antibody substance prepared from the blood of immune persons or animals. When injected into persons exposed to certain infectious diseases, immune globulin can prevent or alter the course of the disease.

WHY ARE COMMUNICABLE DISEASES A SPECIAL PROBLEM IN GROUP SETTINGS FOR YOUNG CHILDREN?

The largest body of information concerning problems associated with communicable diseases in group settings comes from research conducted in day care centers. These facilities house large numbers of children and provide valuable information about the epidemiology, or transmission characteristics of such diseases. However, issues related to communicable diseases in day care centers can be applied to any setting involving groups of young children. Early childhood education classrooms, special preschool programs for handicapped children, special infant centers, and kindergartens are all confronted with the same problems.

THE VULNERABILITY OF THE IMMUNE SYSTEM

Under normal circumstances, the human immune system does not make antibodies prior to birth. Once outside the uterus, newborns are exposed to large numbers of organisms and many are potentially harmful. Fortunately, some of the mother's antibodies cross the placental barrier during pregnancy. Maternal antibodies offer a degree of protection for newborns in the first weeks. Gradually an infant's immune system produces antibodies in response to contact with extrauterine microorganisms. Each time a child's immune system identifies a new, potentially hazardous microorganism, it responds by developing a specific antibody for protection. Eventually, children accumulate a large inventory of antibodies which may offer protection against recurrence of a variety of illnesses. Infants and toddlers get sick frequently, because their repertoire of antibodies is limited.

LARGE POOLS OF VULNERABLE CHILDREN

More than 50 percent of all children in the United States have mothers who work outside the home (Andersen et al., 1986). It is estimated that 11 million children may be enrolled in day care centers by 1990 (Children's Defense Fund, 1986). In Canada, 52 percent of women with children have jobs outside the home, and it is estimated that about 20 percent have some sort of day care arrangements (Ford-Jones et al., 1987). If this trend continues, it is likely that very young children cared for in group settings will be a special source of communicable disease problems. Infants and toddlers in groups are at greater risk for infectious disease than older children. For example, hepatitis outbreaks are more common in centers which accept children under 2 years of age (Child Day Care Infectious Disease Study Group, 1984). Because so many illnesses are spread by direct contact or by the oral-fecal route, diaper changing is the riskiest procedure with respect to transmission of disease. Young children in diapers, children with mouthing behaviors, large numbers of children in a small area, high child-to-caretaker ratio, and limited access to running water or toilet facilities are contributing factors in disease transmission.

SPECIAL GROUPS AT RISK

Handicapped children in general are not at higher risk than nonhandicapped children, but the kind and severity of disabilities may predispose a child to infection. For instance, children with Down syndrome seem to have a higher incidence of respiratory infections, children with cleft palate have frequent ear infections, and children with spina bifida have frequent urinary tract infections. In addition, children with chronic illnesses like leukemia, and children with impaired immune systems are at risk for infectious disease.

PATTERNS OF CONCERN

Concerns of administrators, teachers, care providers, parents, and public health officials can be grouped into four areas (Aronson and Osterholm, 1984). First, there are infections which can cause illness primarily among young children in child care settings (e.g., *Haemophilus influenzae* type b). Second, there are certain infections that equally affect children in child care settings, child care staff, and close family members (e.g., viral diarrhea). Third, there are infections which cause few, if any, symptoms in young children, but can cause serious illness in adult contacts (e.g., hepatitis A). And last, some infections cause mild or no illness in most children or adults, but are potentially serious to unborn children of pregnant contacts. These infections are of special concern to pregnant women and include rubella (German measles), cytomegalovirus (CMV), varicella (chickenpox), herpes, hepatitis B, acquired immunodeficiency syndrome (AIDS), syphilis, and toxoplasmosis.

WHAT ARE PROBLEM DISEASES FOR YOUNG CHILDREN?

Table 4-1 lists diseases which are commonly found or are of special concern in group settings.

The majority of problem illnesses are caused by viruses and bacteria. Most bacterial illnesses can be controlled with antibiotics. Unfortunately this is not true of viral illnesses. Although all of these illnesses are important, some are more serious than others. City, county, and state health agencies maintain lists of diseases which can affect community health and should be reported. *Reportable diseases* are usually grouped into three categories: rare and extremely important diseases that should be reported immediately by telephone (e.g., tuberculosis), common diseases that have a substantial public health impact but do not require urgent reporting (e.g., hepatitis A), and routine infections for which reporting is requested only during outbreaks (e.g., measles). A current list of reportable diseases is available from community health agencies. Administrators, teachers, and other workers in child care should become familiar with disease reporting procedures.

It is also important for professionals to understand their role in the control of communicable disease in group settings. Staff should be alert to symptoms or unusual behaviors which might indicate an illness. After a child returns to a center following an illness, staff should seek information regarding the likelihood of recurrence, transmission, and special precautions to minimize potential transmission. This can be facilitated through good com-

Table 4-1. INFECTIOUS DISEASES IN GROUP SETTINGS

Disease	Mode of Transmission	Causative Agent
Upper respiratory infection*	Respiratory	V
Streptococcal sore throat*	Respiratory	B
Otitis media (ear infection)	Respiratory	V or B
Haemophilus influenzae type b	Respiratory	B
Meningitis	Respiratory	V or B
Tuberculosis	Respiratory	B
Hepatitis A*	Oral-fecal	V
Hepatitis B	Body fluid	V
Hepatitis non-A, non-B	Body fluid	V
Shigella diarrhea*	Oral-fecal	B
Salmonella diarrhea*	Oral-fecal	B
Giardia diarrhea*	Oral-fecal	O
Viral gastroenteritis*	Oral-fecal	V
Impetigo	Direct	B
Ringworm	Direct	F
Scabies*	Direct	O
Herpes simplex (cold sore)	Direct	V
Cytomegalovirus (CMV) infection*	Multiple	V
Chickenpox*	Multiple	V
Head lice*	Direct	O
Pinworms	Oral-fecal	O
Acquired immunodeficiency syndrome (AIDS)	Body fluid	V
Conjunctivitis (pinkeye)	Direct	V or B
Mumps	Respiratory	V
Croup	Respiratory	V
Whooping cough	Respiratory	B
Measles	Respiratory	V
German measles	Respiratory	V
Roseola	Direct	V

V = Virus; B = bacteria; F = fungus; O = other.
* Frequent occurrence in group settings for children.

munication with families, primary health care providers, and public health officials.

Measures for controlling infection are directly related to the mode of transmission. Generally, communicable diseases in group settings are transmitted by respiratory droplet, direct contact, oral-fecal contact, or body fluid contact. It is important to understand that some diseases can be transmitted by more than one mode. For instance, CMV can be transmitted by direct contact, oral-fecal contact, or respiratory droplet.

Information on a variety of illnesses is readily available (see Suggested Reading at the end of this chapter). To illustrate diseases of concern for young children in group settings, their families, and staff, four representative illnesses will be presented. *Upper respiratory infections* will be described because they are representative of infections which are spread primarily by respiratory droplet, and because they are the most common childhood illnesses. *Cytomegalovirus* (CMV) infection will be discussed because of its ability to affect unborn children. Further, CMV is an example of a disease which has several modes of transmission. *Hepatitis A* is representative of diarrheal illness spread by the oral-fecal route. Finally, *AIDS* is an illness spread by intimate contact with blood or other body fluids.

UPPER RESPIRATORY INFECTIONS (COLDS)

Upper respiratory infections are the most common illnesses in young children. In the home, preschoolers have an average of three to eight colds a year (Crosson et al., 1986). Respiratory illness occurs with greatest frequency during the second 6 months of a child's life (Sleator, 1983). It seems logical that the number of colds a child experiences would increase with exposure to other children. However, there are no studies which support this assumption (Crosson et al., 1986).

In very young children *Haemophilus influenzae* type b, commonly referred to as *Hib*, is of special concern. This organism can cause skin infections, joint infections, severe sore throat, pneumonia, or meningitis (an inflammation of the filmy covering of the brain). This is a very uncommon disease, but children under the age of 4 years seem to be at increased risk because they often lack protective antibodies to Hib. Preliminary studies seem to indicate that children in day care centers are at higher risk for Hib than those who stay at home (Fleming et al., 1986). When there is a Hib outbreak in group settings, medical consultants usually advise vaccination or antibiotic treatment of susceptible contacts. Fortunately, treatment can eradicate this infection.

Transmission

There are over 100 microorganisms which can cause respiratory infections. The majority of these organisms are viruses. Although the primary means of transmission is by respiratory droplet, direct contact with infected secretions can also be a route of transmission. Viruses which cause respiratory infections are frequently found on the hands of infected children. Further, viruses can be isolated on approximately 15 percent of objects handled by an ill child. These viruses can survive for up to 48 hr on hard, nonporous surfaces, including plastic toys or cups (Crosson et al., 1986).

Unfortunately, infected children do not display symptoms of a cold (e.g., fever, cough, runny nose) for several days after contact. However, during incubation, children are still contagious. Even after symptoms have subsided, children may continue to shed viral particles for as long as 2 weeks.

Since colds are common and typically mild, and children are frequently infectious before the symptoms of a cold appear, exclusion of a child with colds in order to prevent transmission is usually futile. Many authorities recommend that children who have symptoms but feel well should be allowed to attend school. Those who are too sick to participate in activities should be kept home (Georgetown University Child Development Center, 1986).

Reasonable efforts to lessen transmissibility should be followed. Additional measures might include "cohorting" children. That is, children with obvious colds might be kept together, but separated from asymptomatic children. Education of staff and children about the importance of good hygiene, especially thorough hand washing after nose-blowing is essential.

CYTOMEGALOVIRUS (CMV)

CMV is a member of the herpes group of viruses. The other members of this group are *herpes simplex* type 1 (cold sores and fever blisters), *herpes simplex* type 2 (genital herpes), *Epstein-Barr* virus (infectious mononucleosis), and *varicella-zoster* (chickenpox).

CMV is the cause of a common viral infection that is usually harmless. Research indicates that antibodies to CMV can be found in approximately 40 percent of children in the United States under the age of 6 years (Evans, 1982). This percentage may vary in other countries. In all countries, it appears that most adults have been infected with CMV. Generally, adults and children who become infected with CMV remain well or have only mild symptoms. Most CMV infections are *asymptomatic* making detection and prevention extremely difficult.

Formerly it was thought that CMV infection was uniformly associated with severe illness of the newborn, and carried a high probability of death or marked damage to the central nervous system. Although CMV infection can result in devastating damage, most infected children show no signs, symptoms, or long-term effects of the disease. Typically, a positive antibody test is the only evidence of infection with CMV (Evans, 1982).

Children who contract CMV infection prior to birth are said to have congenital cytomegalic inclusion disease. One percent or less of all infants born in the United States will be infected but most will be perfectly normal. Of this 1 percent, only 10 to 15 percent will develop a disability of some sort. When severe damage occurs, it seems to be associated with first, or primary infec-

Figure 4-1. Cytomegalovirus (CMV) infection during pregnancy.

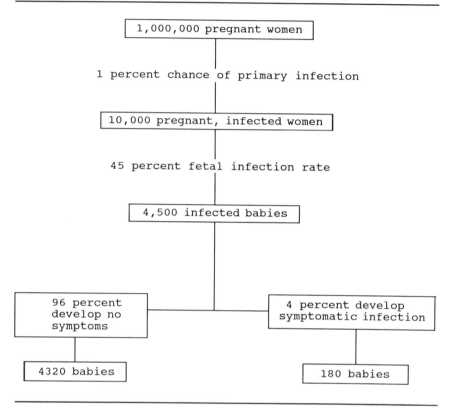

tions. Since the majority of adult women have already had CMV infection before becoming pregnant, only the minority will be at some risk. It has been shown that there is only a 1 percent chance of a pregnant women developing a primary infection (Gehrz, 1984). Even when an infection is acquired during pregnancy, transmission to the fetus occurs in only 45 percent (Interview with Sergio Stagno: Isolation precautions for patients with cytomegalovirus infection, 1982). Another way of looking at these statistics is demonstrated in Figure 4-1. For unknown reasons, women with secondary infections during pregnancy rarely give birth to severely affected infants. Although the risk of transmitting CMV prenatally appears to be small, it is especially important for women of child-bearing age to observe good personal hygiene, especially hand washing (Gehrz, 1984).

Transmission

CMV can be transmitted via body fluids, including breast milk, and across the placenta to fetuses. CMV is believed to be widespread. Close physical contact seems to be required for transmission. Urine and saliva are thought to be the major sources of infection. In child care settings, CMV is most likely to be transmitted by contact with feces, urine, and saliva.

CMV transmission from an infected child to a pregnant staff member or parent is a concern. Although definitive research is necessary, studies of women who work with CMV infected children suggest that these women are no more likely to acquire infection than are other women in the community (Andersen et al., 1986). To minimize transmission of CMV, the following guidelines have been recommended. First, wash hands frequently and thoroughly, especially after diapering. Second, dispose of diapers properly. Third, disinfect diaper-changing areas, shared toys, and other articles which may be mouthed frequently. And last, provide educational programs for staff, students, and parents (Andersen et al., 1986).

According to the Centers for Disease Control (CDC), routine screening of pregnant women in "high-exposure" areas is not indicated because specific risks have not been established. Further, testing facilities are not readily available and the significance of a single antibody test is difficult to interpret. It is not known whether the risk of primary infection could be reduced by transferring antibody-negative women to assignments involving no contact with potentially infected infants and children (Centers for Disease Control, 1985). To be cautious, employers should consider a program of antibody testing for employees. Results could be used by employees and their physicians for interpretation and discussion of work assignment options. Women who have children in group settings should probably be tested for CMV antibody if they anticipate pregnancy because it has been shown that young children can acquire the infection in group settings and transmit it to either parent (Pass et al., 1986).

Currently there is no CMV vaccine available; however, research is encouraging. When a vaccine is developed it may be recommended for use by all antibody-negative women of childbearing age.

HEPATITIS A

Viral hepatitis is an infectious disease which affects the liver. Viruses that cause hepatitis are classified as hepatitis A, hepatitis B, and hepatitis non-A, non-B viruses. At the present time only hepatitis A has been determined to be a significant problem in child care settings.

The severity of hepatitis A varies with age. About 75 percent of infected children will feel sick, and the majority will also experience nausea, fever, and diarrhea. Only about 5 to 10 percent will acquire a yellowish caste of the skin or eyes, called *jaundice*. Among adults, however, the disease is more easily recognized since about 75 percent will become jaundiced. The illness lasts from 2 to 8 weeks and tends to be milder in children. Almost all those infected recover with no disability (Hadler and McFarland, 1986). Unlike CMV, the hepatitis A virus does not seem to cause any special problems for the unborn child of a woman who is pregnant.

Transmission

Hepatitis A is spread primarily by the oral-fecal route, while hepatitis B and hepatitis non-A, non-B are transmitted by blood, or blood-associated secretions, contaminated needles, sexual contacts, and infected blood transfusions. Hepatitis B and hepatitis non-A, non-B are *not* transmitted via the oral-fecal route. Hepatitis A can be spread by direct person-to-person contact, by contaminated food or water, or by contaminated objects. These modes of transmission are identical to those for other diarrheal illnesses such as shigellosis, salmonellosis, giardiasis, and viral gastroenteritis. Therefore, every unusual diarrheal illness must be properly diagnosed.

Hepatitis A seems to be very contagious, and outbreaks of several cases in an institution are common. There are several important factors about hepatitis A which should be recognized. Outbreaks are more common in facilities with young, diapered children, and affected children often have few symptoms. Children can spread hepatitis A easily to other children and adults, and the illness tends to be more severe and last longer in older children and adults. Hepatitis A has a very long incubation period, averaging 30 days, and the virus is shed in feces for as much as 2 weeks before symptoms of illness, if any, appear (Sleator, 1983). For these reasons the presence of hepatitis A may become apparent only when affected adults discover they have children at the same center.

Hepatitis A can be detected by laboratory tests in the absence of symptoms. If a child feels ill, complains of frequent abdominal pain, has poor appetite, low-grade fever, and then develops dark, tea-colored urine or light clay-colored feces, hepatitis A should be suspected and reported to the child's parents immediately. If hepatitis A is confirmed, local public health officials should be notified in order to control the outbreak. One measure used for control is injection of a substance called *immune globulin* or *gamma globulin*. This is a concentration of antibodies against the hepatitis A virus. This is an example of *passive immunization*, as described in Chapter 2. In day care centers with children under the age of 2 years experiencing an outbreak of hepatitis A, immune globulin is recommended for all children and employees, and in some instances for household contacts of all children under the age of 3 years (Child Day Care Infectious Disease Study Group, 1984). In addition to practicing good hygiene, staff should report all diarrheal illness. Failure to do so may lead to delay in diagnosis and control of a serious outbreak.

ACQUIRED IMMUNODEFICIENCY SYNDROME (AIDS)

As previously described, many microorganisms prefer to invade specific body sites or tissues. For instance, some organisms prefer the nose and throat areas, causing colds; other organisms prefer the intestinal tract, causing stomach upset and diarrhea. Normally, any kind of infection, regardless of the location, will cause a quick and effective response from the body's natural defenses, or immune system. A large portion of the immune system is composed of a specific type of white blood cell, called lymphocytes. These cells are attacked by the human immunodeficiency virus (HIV), which causes an illness called acquired immunodeficiency syndrome (AIDS). It is easy to see why AIDS is such a difficult and worrisome disease. The system in our bodies which normally protects us from a wide variety of diseases is paralysed when attacked by this peculiar virus. AIDS victims are ill, not because of the direct effects of the virus, but because the body cannot defend itself against a large number of organisms which ordinarily are unable to cause illness.

The origins of HIV are still unknown, but there is evidence that the present global epidemic, a pandemic, began in the mid- to late 1970s. The disease was not recognized, however, until 1981, and the virus was not discovered until 1983 (Gong and Rudnick, 1987). In a report by the World Health Organization, it was estimated that as of summer, 1988, there were as many as 250,000 cases of AIDS worldwide, and that there are likely to be between 5 to 10 million persons infected (Mann and Chin, 1988). The problem is compounded by an extremely long incubation period. It appears there may be many persons infected with HIV who have no symptoms. Much important information about HIV and AIDS is known. Modes of transmission are well documented. Special groups who are at high risk for HIV have been identified. Reliable screening and diagnostic tests have been developed and are available and reliable. AIDS appears to be difficult to contract. And avoidance of risky behaviors has been shown to be an effective prevention strategy.

Transmission

In studying the transmission characteristics of HIV and AIDS, scientists have determined that the virus is spread only by contact with blood, semen, vaginal secretions, and possibly breast milk. HIV is spread during sexual contact, needle sharing, and is directly transmitted from mother to child prior to birth, during delivery, or after birth. The virus can also be transmitted through transfusion of infected blood or blood products. Initially, it was thought that transmission by heterosexual contact was unlikely, but recent information suggest that this assumption may have been incorrect. It is now well-known, however, that casual family contact such as hugging, kissing, sharing cooking utensils, dishes, food, and toilet facilities does not result in transmission of the virus. And it has been demonstrated that HIV is *not* spread by the oral-fecal route or by droplet (Silverman and Waddell, 1987).

AIDS affects both men and women, but of all the reported cases, less than 20 percent are women (Gong and Rudnick, 1987). One half of women affected with AIDS are intravenous drug abusers, or sexual partners of men from high-risk groups (intravenous drug abusers, bisexual men, and hemophiliacs who have had repeated blood transfusions).

As previously mentioned, HIV can be passed from mother to child prior to birth. It is estimated that the risk of a newborn becoming infected from its mother is about 50 percent, and the risk seems to increase with each successive pregnancy (Gong and Rudnick, 1987).

There are two issues which must be addressed in the care of HIV-infected children in group settings. First, affected children may be at greater risk for acquiring an infection from a classmate than of infecting others. Second, the degree of potential for an infected child transmitting the virus to others must be considered (MacDonald, Danila, and Osterholm, 1986). The Committee on Infectious Diseases of the American Academy of Pediatrics (1987) has published recommendations for the care of infected children in group settings. Recommendations include a restricted environment for children who lack bowel or bladder control, who drool, have uncoverable skin lesions, or whose behaviors may increase the risk of transmission (e.g., biting). According to MacDonald and colleagues (1986), decisions regarding placement of HIV-infected children should be made on a case-by-case basis, by evaluating potential risks to others, and the infected child.

It would be reasonable to test all children at risk for acquiring HIV infection before admission to a group setting (MacDonald et al., 1986). Diagnostic screening should be performed in children who received blood transfusions between 1978 and 1985, children who have been sexually abused, and children who have been born to HIV-positive mothers or to mothers who are themselves at risk. In situations where an HIV-infected child is skilled at toileting, practices appropriate hygiene, and has no oozing or uncovered lesions, admission to a public group setting is appropriate and does not appear to pose a significant threat to other students or staff (Committee on Infectious Diseases: American Academy of Pediatrics, 1987). Child care centers should intensify educational programs for students, parents, and staff about infectious diseases in general, and HIV infection specifically.

SUMMARY

Immaturity of the immune system in infants and young children makes them especially susceptible to infectious organisms. Gatherings of children in group settings virtually assures a greater chance of coming into contact with others who have symptomatic or asymptomatic infections.

Most infections are either bacterial or viral and are spread by known modes of transmission. These modes are classified as respiratory droplet, direct contact, oral-fecal, or blood and body fluid exposure with injury. Upper respiratory infections, CMV infection, hepatitis A, and AIDS are presented as examples.

Some infectious diseases of children can also affect adults and have very serious consequences for the unborn child of a pregnant woman. It is therefore very important that information about infectious diseases in group settings be available to staff workers and parents, as well as program administrators.

SUGGESTED READING

Andersen, R. D., Bale, J. F., Blackman, J. A., and Murph, J. R. (1986). *Infections in children: A sourcebook for educators and child care providers*. Rockville, MD: Aspen.

Committee on Infectious Diseases: American Academy of Pediatrics (1987). Health guidelines for the attendance in day-care and foster care settings of children infected with human immunodeficiency virus. *Pediatrics, 79*, 466–471.

Crosson, F. J., Black, S. B., Trumpp, C. E., Grossman, M., Lé, C. T., and Yeager, A. S. (1986). Infections in day care centers. *Current Problems in Pediatrics, 16*, 122–184.

Gehrz, R. C. (1984). CMV: *Diagnosis, prevention and treatment*. St. Paul, MN: Children's Hospital of St. Paul.

Sleator, E. K. (1983). *Infectious diseases in day care*. Urbana, IL: Clearinghouse on Elementary and Early Childhood Education, University of Illinois.

CHAPTER 5

Recommendations

IMPORTANT TERMS

Disinfectant

A disinfectant is a chemical sanitizing agent, usually a liquid, which inactivates or kills microorganisms.

Bleach

Bleach is a common laundering agent containing chlorine, which can be used as a disinfectant when diluted properly.

Universal precautions   Universal precautions is the concept of performing a task as if all the recipients of the service were infected, even in the absence of signs or symptoms of illness.

SCOPE OF SERVICES

It is anticipated that challenges associated with communicable diseases and group settings for young children will exist for many years. Solving problems related to infectious disease control in child care centers will require cooperative efforts of parents, educators, child care providers, health care professionals, private industry, and federal, state, and local governments. For now, it is imperative that adults concerned with the health of young children in group settings learn how to minimize the risk of transmitting communicable diseases in children's centers.

WHAT POLICIES SHOULD BE DEVELOPED?

ENVIRONMENTAL

Settings for groups of young children will vary from community to community and be affected by the resources available. Day care is often provided in churches, schools, private homes, and businesses. Space is frequently modified for children's activities, and leased by care providers. Guidelines can be obtained from professional organizations (e.g., the National Association for the Education of Young Children; see Appendix for resources regarding recommended amounts of space per child, number of lavatories, food preparation facilities, class size, and size of playground area). However, in the United States, federal statutory standards for child care practices are lacking (Aronson and Osterholm, 1984). Indeed, at the present time "there are no federal regulations directed specifically to the general health of children in day care" (Committee on Early Childhood, Adoption and Dependent Care: American Academy of Pediatrics, 1987, p. 116).

The American Academy of Pediatrics offers the following issues for policy consideration in establishing healthful environments for young children in day care: Classrooms should be large enough to accommodate a wide variety of activities without crowding; ventilation should be adequate; temperature control should be easy; bathrooms should be readily accessible to children and staff; there should be separate bathrooms for workers involved with food preparation; floors and walls should be made of materials that can be easily cleaned and disinfected; and food preparation areas should be set apart from classroom areas (Committee on Early Childhood, Adoption and Dependent Care: American Academy of Pediatrics, 1987). It is difficult to find facilities which lend themselves easily to these principles, and conversion of an existing space to accommodate these recommendations may be physically or financially difficult. Compromises are inevitable. When faced with difficult space issues, input from local public health officials is essential.

STAFFING

Recruitment of well-trained staff members may be a problem. Many potential applicants have had no training or experience. Although most workers have some education beyond high school, many are paid minimum wage with few fringe benefits. Salaries are frequently below the poverty level. Because of low salary levels it is not unusual to have a 50 percent turnover of staff every 2 years (Kendall et al., 1986). With increased national awareness of child abuse in children's centers (Hollingsworth, 1986), it seems critical that prospective employees receive background checks and adequate supervision when caring for children. Additionally, a pre-employment medical evaluation, which specifically addresses health issues related to child care, should be required. At a minimum, health examinations should include a medical history of infectious diseases, past or present physical impairments, and comments regarding temperament and emotional stability. In addition, immunizations should be current. Antibody testing could provide information regarding exposure to specific diseases. If performed, antibody testing should address antibody levels for measles, German measles, mumps, and polio. In some instances herpes, cytomegalovirus (CMV), hepatitis, and acquired immunodeficiency syndrome (AIDS) antibody levels should also be measured. Day care directors should be aware that any information obtained by a physician as the result of a medical evaluation is confidential and may not be released until approved by the employee in writing. This information should remain confidential when transferred to an employee's file.

CLASS GROUPINGS

Generally, children should be segregated by age, toileting status, and infection status. *Infants and toddlers* are usually not toilet trained and more likely to spread infectious microorganisms found in saliva, urine, and feces. They should be separated from *well children* who are toilet trained. *Children who become ill* while at the care center should be kept apart from infants and toddlers and older children who are not ill. It is likely that whatever microorganism is responsible for an illness contracted by a child in a day care center has already been spread to several other persons before symptoms appear. Nevertheless, it makes good sense to separate ill children until they have been picked up by their parents or a medical evaluation has been performed.

The U.S. Congress declared a policy of educating handicapped children with nonhandicapped "to the maximum extent appropriate" (Weiner and Hume, 1987). A similar policy recommendation was offered by the Centers for Disease Control (1985). With the exception of children who exhibit problem behaviors (e.g., biting, spitting), it is anticipated that handicapped and nonhandicapped children will continue to be grouped together in educational or day care settings (Guralnick, 1978).

ADMINISTRATION

A written policy manual is the structural backbone of an early childhood education or child care program. Policy manuals should contain information regarding administrative organization, aims and objectives of the center, and specific strategies for achieving those objectives. Because it is well-known that communicable diseases are inevitable in group settings for young children, policies related to health care should be included. State and local regulations, health consultants, sick child care, and exclusion of ill children should be clearly delineated.

State Regulations

The main mechanism for regulation of day care is licensing by state governments. Licensing is usually a function of state social service agencies, although in a few states health agencies performs this task (Morgan et al., 1986). Regulations vary with regard to infection control. For instance, in some states any child who is ill must be sent home. Some states leave exclusion decisions to officials in individual centers. Other states have no regulations relating to exclusion of ill children (Shapiro, Kuritsky, and Potter, 1986). In states with minimal regulatory control, varied interpretations are allowed with a "great likelihood of poor health practices" (Committee on Early Childhood, Adoption and Dependent Care: American Academy of Pediatrics, 1987, p. 117). In some instances compliance with current standards appears to be limited or ignored by both parents and care providers (Kendall et al., 1986).

Most states have regulations, albeit varied, for the following: hand washing, employee health examinations, personal toilet articles, medical record-keeping, admission procedures, isolation for illness, return to care after illness, notification of parents concerning outbreaks of communicable diseases, reportable diseases, admission or exclusion of mildly ill children, infant care, adult-to-infant ratios, group size, health consultants, health policies, staff training, and parent education (Morgan et al., 1986). It is important for administrators to be familiar with regulatory practices in their state. Until a national standard of child care practices is established, professionals can lobby for regulations based on scientific fact and which are uniformly acceptable. Because restrictive regulations tend to increase child care costs, care should be taken to advocate development of state standards which ensure access by all children, regardless of economic resources.

Health Consultant

Due to the frequency of illness in group settings for young children, and importance of rapid recognition and management of infectious diseases, each center should consider retention of a health care consultant. Pediatricians, pediatric nurse-practitioners, family nurse-practitioners, and public health nurses are logical sources of consultative services. Family practitioners with pediatric experience can also serve as health care consultants to programs. Practitioners should not be hired as "school doctors" to diagnose and treat sick children, but should serve in a consultative capacity for communicable disease oversight. Health care consultants can perform the following tasks:

Evaluation of student admission applications. Children should have physical examinations performed by their primary physicians as an admission requirement. Health care consultants should review health records in order to identify past health problems which might affect classroom or teacher assignment, and specific problems which might warrant special attention. This is especially important for handicapped children who may have congenital infections or impaired immune systems. Immunization records should be reviewed to ensure that current guidelines are met.

Evaluation of prospective employees. Medical histories and results of pre-employment physical examinations of prospective employees should be carefully reviewed prior to employment. Immunization records should be evaluated for completeness. As previously noted, antibody testing for previous exposure to certain diseases should be performed and evaluated. Antibody status could be especially valuable to the employee if pregnancy is contemplated.

Health policy recommendations. Health care consultants can provide recommendations for policies related to health issues. Health focussed policies may include disease control, sick child care, exclusion, first aid, and management of communicable disease outbreaks. It is recommended that employees receive annual medical evaluations and tuberculosis skin testing. Some authorities also advise annual influenza vaccination (Sleator, 1983).

Educational programs. Staff should have regular inservice educational programs. Health issues should be addressed, including communicable disease transmission, communicable disease prevention, and recognition of illness in children. In situations where a center provides care for ill children, educational programs should be more frequent and probably more detailed. Similar educational programs could be tailored for parents. After consultation with the physician of an ill child, medical consultants might offer advice to staff on a case-by-case basis.

Monitoring functions. Health consultants should monitor occurrences of communicable diseases based on regular reports from the child care center for purposes of reporting to local health agencies. In turn, any public health recommendations could be made directly to the health consultant. After meeting with center administrators and staff, consultants could then assist with development of plans to control, prevent, or monitor specific communicable diseases.

Liaison functions. Contact with health care providers serving children enrolled in a center should be a regular duty of a health care consultant. In this way the entire medical community could participate in disease prevention issues. Health consultants could organize *health advisory committees*, comprised of parents, physicians, public health nurses, local public health department representatives, building inspectors, and consumer safety representatives (Committee on Early Childhood, Adoption and Dependent

Care: American Academy of Pediatrics, 1987) to serve as advisors for health-related issues.

Management of outbreaks. In the event of a serious outbreak of communicable disease, it is important for health consultants to gather and interpret relevant medical information for purposes of making specific recommendations. For example, when an outbreak of hepatitis A occurs in a center, a health consultant would be expected to notify local public health officials, assist local health officials with plans for administration of immune globulin to contacts, notify parents, notify other physicians in the community, and put into effect any other measures which might be necessary to control the outbreak.

Sick Child Care and Exclusion Policy

There appears to be no evidence that children prolong their recovery by attending school while mildly ill if staffing is adequate in a day care center (Shapiro et al., 1986). Many communicable diseases can be transmitted before symptoms appear. Therefore, exclusion policies may not be effective in preventing contagion. If mildly ill children can be cared for without compromising the health and care of others, exclusion may not be warranted (Shapiro et al., 1986). There are a few diseases which *require* that a child be excluded from the care setting (Georgetown University Child Development Center, 1986). The most common illnesses that appear on exclusion lists are *diarrhea, pinkeye, head lice, contagious skin conditions, persistent sore throat, chickenpox*, and *undiagnosed fevers*. Some exclusion policies include: meningococcal meningitis, *Haemophilus influenzae* type b (Hib) disease, hepatitis, and AIDS or human immunodeficiency virus (HIV) infection under certain circumstances. Sick child care policy and exclusion policy should be clearly written and distributed to parents on their first visit.

A written policy regarding care of children who become sick is crucial. The language should be simple, direct, and easily understood by parents. Creation of this kind of policy can be an arduous task. It should address state or local public health regulations, space and personnel requirements, and recommendations from the health consultant. When possible the policy should reflect awareness of the expense for home care for sick children, parental leave policies related to ill children, and the unpredictable nature of communicable diseases in young children. There is no standard policy that is acceptable to all providers of child care because of differing physical facilities, number and qualifications of personnel, and needs of parents being served.

It is likely that child care centers will continue to feel pressure to provide facilities for sick children (Jordan, 1986). Caring for sick children involves challenges. For example, staffing requirements, administration of medications, medical supervision, appropriate cohorting of sick children, and public safety must be considered. Fortunately, liability problems associated with communicable disease in child care centers have been few (Sleator, 1983). Most children harboring infectious microorganisms are contagious and have already spread their infection before they develop symptoms. Nevertheless certain communicable diseases do have potentially serious public health consequences, and require reporting to public health authorities. Policies related to sick child care should be formulated based on center needs, family issues, and child needs. Each center should develop a list of diseases *and* symptoms that require exclusion from the center until the contagious stage is passed.

Food Preparation and Storage

The American Academy of Pediatrics recommends hiring a professional sanitarian to review food handling practices and equipment (Committe on Early Childhood, Adoption and Dependent Care: American Academy of Pediatrics, 1987). Consultation by a professional sanitarian should be sought even if state and local regulations do not address this issue. Policies relating to food storage, preparation, transport, and clean-up procedures could be reviewed by a health care consultant. Of particular concern are policies related to handling of infant formula and commercial baby foods.

Disease Control

Although illness is inevitable in child care settings, good hygiene can contribute to reductions in frequency and duration of communicable diseases. To this end, certain procedures should be followed routinely. These procedures should be delineated in policy manuals after careful analysis by a health consultant. Hygienic measures specific to each route of transmission should be clearly listed: oral-fecal, respiratory, direct contact, and contact with body fluids. Further, disease prevention policies should be updated frequently as information becomes available.

EDUCATIONAL PROGRAMS

Due to the frequency of illness in young children, communicable disease transmission is inevitable. Parents should be informed of the possibility of illness as a result of group contacts. It is also important to provide parents with information regarding each family's responsibility for informing center staff of symptoms or illness in their child. When enrolling children in a child care or educational program, parents should be provided with informative materials related to communicable disease transmission in group settings for young children. Further, ongoing parent education programs addressing communicable disease issues are advisable.

Prior to employment, staff should receive information regarding infectious disease control policies. In addition, they should be assured that policies were developed with the welfare of children, families, *and* staff in mind. Staff inservice sessions should address health and safety concerns whenever they arise.

WHAT ARE SPECIFIC RECOMMENDATIONS FOR PREVENTION OR CONTROL OF COMMUNICABLE DISEASE ?

CENTER DESIGN

Research regarding communicable disease transmission in child care facilities suggests that readily available hand-washing facilities, segregation of children by age, and use of easily cleaned surfaces contribute to disease reduction (Petersen and Bressler, 1986). Designs for new facilities and modification of existing structures should address health concerns for staff and children. Local building code requirements and financial constraints often present challenges to development of a healthful environment. Also, finding an architect or space designer who is knowledgeable about space requirements and public health problems can be difficult. However, the long-term benefits of adequate planning relative to a healthy environment will have multiple benefits.

Petersen and Bressler (1986) suggest designing child care centers around a central core. Food preparation and storage, janitorial facilities, and toilet facilities could be clustered in this centralized location. Offices and conference rooms could be planned for proximity to the front entrance. Space for children's activities should be divided between rooms for infant and toddler care and "open" spaces for older children. Infant and toddler rooms and food handling areas should be separated by walls from other areas in the building. Kitchen surfaces should be chosen for cleanability and durability. Use of stainless steel sinks, laminated plastic surfaces and cabinets, vinyl floor sheeting, and washable lead-free wall paint are recommended. Food handlers should have separate bathroom and hand-washing facilities with pedal-operated sinks, liquid soap containers, and paper towel dispensers.

Floors in areas used by children can be carpeted or tiled. Since tile is more easily cleaned, eating should be restricted to tiled areas. Diaper-changing areas in infant or toddler rooms should be close to running water and restricted from use for other purposes. Changing tables and shelves should be covered with laminated plastic for easy cleaning. Toddler rooms should have appropriately sized toilet and handwashing fixtures. Staff hand-washing facilities should be readily accessible and have knee-operated water controls, liquid soap containers, and paper towel dispensers. Additional considerations include lighting, ventilation, furnishings, drinking fountains, and playground equipment.

There are many other acceptable design plans, but all should address health and safety issues for children, families, and staff. It is also important to note that facility planning is worthless unless good hygiene is practiced routinely.

HYGIENE

Creation of a sterile environment for children and staff is not likely. By nature, social activities for children will involve transmission of microorganisms from one child or adult to another. As educators and child care providers strive to provide safe and healthful environments for young children, certain procedures should be performed as a matter of routine. They could be called the 11 commandments of cleanliness and disinfection;

    I. Wear clean smocks and change daily.
    II. Wash play surfaces and toys daily.
    III. Sweep and mop floors at the end of each day.
    IV. Clean walls weekly.
    V. Collect trash in tied, plastic bags, and dispose of daily.
    VI. Collect soiled cloth diapers in sealed plastic bags and send home for laundering.

Cleaning and disinfecting surfaces is a five-stage procedure:

    VII. Wear gloves to clean spills of body fluids.
    VIII. Wipe up visible soil with paper towels.
    IX. Wash the area with soap or detergent and water.
    X. Rinse the area with clean water.
    XI. Disinfect the area.

Commercial disinfectant or a solution of ¼ cup of liquid household bleach in 1 gallon of water may be used. The area can be left to air-dry, or after 20 minutes can be rinsed with clean water and then left to air-dry. This concentration of bleach will inactivate hepatitis A virus, HIV, and many other disease-producing microorganisms. A similar concentration of bleach should be available in a pump spray bottle for application to small, or hard-to-reach surfaces. The bottles and storage containers of bleach or water solutions and commercial disinfectants should be clearly labeled and out of reach of children.

Hand-washing reminder posters should be placed in each lavatory. Food preparation and service should be provided by workers who are free of skin lesions, and who have no responsibilities for the care of infants or toddlers.

HAND WASHING

A review of the literature related to communicable diseases and young children in group settings will undoubtedly reveal a common theme. *Hand washing is probably the single most effective procedure for prevention of transmission of communicable diseases* (Committee on Early Childhood, Adoption and Dependent Care: American Academy of Pediatrics, 1987).

Hand washing should be performed by child care providers on arrival at the center, before eating or drinking, after using the toilet, after diaper changing, and after contact with an infected child or infected items such as tissues, mouthed toys, or eating utensils. After removing any jewelry, the hands should be washed with adequate soap (preferably liquid), under running water, using friction, and should cover all skin surfaces to at least the midpoint of the lower arm. After thorough rinsing, hands should be dried with paper towels. Hand washing at a sink equipped with knee or foot pedals is preferable. When this is not possible, it is acceptable to turn on faucets with "dirty" hands, wash and dry hands, and then turn off faucets with paper towels (see Figure 5-1).

The faucet fixture can be sprayed with disinfectant after hand washing. If performed properly and as frequently as recommended, many workers will develop dry, cracked, and chapped hands. These breaks in the skin can be sources of entry of microorganisms into the body. Preventive measures such as the liberal use of skin creams and lotions are therefore recommended.

DIAPERING AND TOILETING

Diaper changing is a high-risk procedure for contamination of the child, caretaker, and environment (Child Day Care Infectious Disease Study Group, 1984). The use of *universal precautions* is appropriate for care providers who are responsible for infants and toddlers. The concept of universal precautions means performing a task as if all the recipients of the service are infected. Since there are so many communicable diseases which are asymp-

Figure 5-1. Hand-washing procedures. (Adapted from Georgetown University Child Development Center [1986]. *Health in day care: A manual for day care providers.* Washington, DC: Author. Reprinted by permission.)

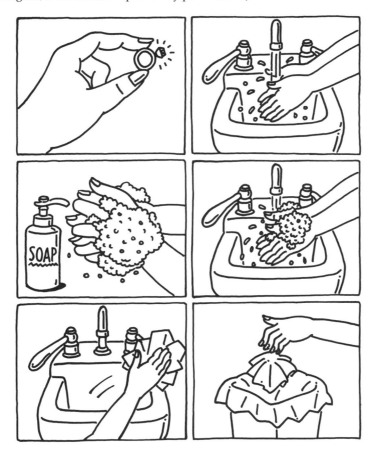

tomatic, infectious in their incubation period, or involve organisms "shedding," it makes sense to use precautions for all children. In the context of diapering and toileting, universal precautions involve procedures that would be used if every child were known to be infected with microorganisms which are transmitted in stool or urine. Disposable latex or plastic gloves could be used. Disposable gloves are expensive, but, thicker "dishwashing" rubber gloves could be used and reused after washing and disinfecting in the manner described previously. Diaper changes should occur in designated areas that are separate from food preparation and serving areas, that have easily cleaned surfaces, and that are within easy reach of a specific sink.

The changing surface should be covered with a disposable covering which is discarded after one use. Contaminated paper products should be disposed of in sealed plastic bags. The changing surface should be washed and disinfected after every procedure. Soiled diapers should be placed in plastic bags and stored in covered trash cans. Soiled clothing should also be placed in plastic bags, sealed, and stored in a covered container until it can be picked up by the parents for laundering at home. Finally, before returning to the classroom from the toilet or diapering area, both care providers and children should have freshly washed hands.

BODY FLUID SPILLS

It is relatively common for young children to have bloody noses or occasional small cuts which bleed. Children may also spit, vomit, or have toileting accidents. Because some microorganisms are spread through these body fluids, thorough clean-up of blood, vomitus, mucus, urine, and feces should occur immediately following an incident. Again, universal precautions are appropriate for cleaning up body fluid spills. The use of thick rubber gloves is advisable. Initially, spills should be wiped up with paper towels which are then discarded. The area should then be washed or mopped with soap or detergent and rinsed. Disinfection, as previously described, should follow.

OTHER HEALTH ISSUES

In addition to hygiene, other potential problems should be addressed. Consideration should be given to development of policies and inservice education regarding routine health screening, child development, behavior management, nutrition, education of children with special problems, and first-aid procedures. Furthermore, employers should have liberal sick leave policies to avoid having staff care for children when they are ill. It follows that substitute staff should be readily available.

Even the most vigilant efforts will not prevent all illness. When an outbreak occurs, parents should be notified promptly. Informative materials should be prepared for distribution in the event of an outbreak. Excellent examples of parent information sheets can be found in *Health in day care: A manual for day care providers* (Georgetown University Child Development Center, 1986).

SUMMARY

No amount of planning, money, scientific research, or design will eliminate infectious diseases from child care centers. It has been demonstrated that attention to certain general and specific concepts will decrease the incidence and severity of infectious diseases in group settings of young children. To this end, setting design, staffing, policy development, and educational programs can be effective in preventing or limiting the spread of communicable diseases.

Recommendations for any group setting involving young children include development of cleaning and disinfecting procedures, hand-washing procedures, diapering and toileting procedures, procedures for management of body fluid spills, and procedures for disposal of soiled materials. Care providers should have a thorough knowledge of these techniques as well as awareness of other factors influencing child health.

SUGGESTED READING

Andersen, R. D., Bale, J. F., Blackman, J. A., and Murph, J. R. (1986). *Infections in children: A sourcebook for educators and child care providers*. Rockville, MD: Aspen.

Committee on Early Childhood, Adoption and Dependent Care: American Academy of Pediatrics (1987). *Health in day care: A manual for health professionals*. Elk Grove Village, IL: American Academy of Pediatrics.

Georgetown University Child Development Center (1986). *Health in day care: A manual for day care providers*. Washington, DC: Author.

Sleator, E. K. (1983). *Infectious diseases in day care*. Urbana, IL: Clearinghouse on Elementary and Early Childhood Education, University of Illinois.

U. S. Department of Health and Human Services (1984). *What you should know about contagious diseases in the day care setting*. Washington, DC: U. S. Government Printing Office.

CHAPTER 6

Legal Issues

IMPORTANT TERMS*

Defendant	A defendant is the "person defending or denying; party against whom relief or recovery is sought in an action or suit..." (p. 377).
In loco parentis	A person who serves "in the place of a parent; instead of a parent" (p. 708) is said to be in loco parentis.
Liability	A person or organization which bears responsibility "for a possible or actual loss" (p. 823) is said to have "liability for their actions or inactions."
Libel	Libelous acts are those in which defamation "expressed by print, writing, pictures, or signs... that is injurious to the reputation of another" (p. 824) occurs.
Malpractice	Misconduct by a professional or an unreasonable lack of skill (p. 836) is known as malpractice.
Negligence	"The doing of some act which a person of ordinary prudence would not have done under similar circumstances or failure to do what a person of ordinary prudence would have done under similar circumstances" (pp. 930–931) is considered negligence.
Plaintiff	"A person who brings an action...the party who complains" (p. 1,035) is known as the plaintiff.
Slander	"The speaking of base and defamatory words tending to prejudice another in his reputation" (p. 1,245) is considered slander.
Tort	Tort law is a "private or civil wrong or injury... for which the court will provide a remedy in the form of an action for damages" (p. 1,335).

*Page references are to Black (1979).

WHAT LIABILITY ISSUES MIGHT BE RELATED TO COMMUNICABLE DISEASES AND GROUP SETTINGS FOR YOUNG CHILDREN?

Almost anyone can be sued. Car owners and home owners usually have insurance coverage for protection against possible lawsuits related to accidental injury. In today's litigation-conscious society, prudent people plan ahead to minimize risks related to lawsuits.

To date, there has been little litigation in response to injury or illness associated with communicable disease transmission in group settings for young children (Sleator, 1983). However, it seems wise to consider legal issues related to communicable diseases and young children. In doing so, it is hoped that a variety of strategies for minimizing risks associated with transmission of communicable diseases will be examined, considered, and implemented.

NEGLIGENCE AND MALPRACTICE

Stevenson, Sterne, and Stephens (1986) have suggested that *negligence would be the most likely issue addressed in potential litigation following the outbreak of an infectious disease.* Underlying the principle of negligence are four basic assumptions: There was (1) a duty to conform to accepted standards of conduct; (2) a failure to meet accepted standards, also known as "a breach of duty"; (3) "proximate cause," a reasonable causal relationship between the damage to the client and the breach; and (4) actual damage or illness. If a negligent act is committed by a professional, a doctor, or teacher, the term *malpractice* is used (VanBiervliet and Sheldon-Wildgen, 1981).

For a staff member to be negligent, there would have to be a clear duty to conform to accepted standards and practices, or a failure to conform to accepted standards and practices, a causal relationship between the failure to perform and an illness or injury, and an actual injury or illness. If litigation was based on negligence or malpractice, this would be especially pertinent to teachers and caretakers, due to the concept of *in loco parentis* (Black, 1979). Adults who care for or teach children are charged with a "parent's rights, duties and responsibilities," and considered in loco parentis. This establishes clear responsibility for a child's welfare (Brown, 1984).

When a person responsible for a child's care fails to act in accordance with established standards and practices, the question of malpractice or liability could be raised. For example, if a teacher was aware that a student with behavior problems was a carrier of hepatitis and permitted unsupervised interactions with other children resulting in infection by one or more children, a lawsuit might ensue. This seems unlikely, of course, but cautious administrators, teachers, or child care workers should take care to provide the safest environment possible and routinely intervene when a child's safety might be endangered.

VIOLATION OF LAWS OR REGULATIONS RELATED TO YOUNG CHILDREN AND GROUP SETTINGS

There is great variability between states with respect to laws and regulations governing the education and care of young children in group settings. Some states have progressive legislation which limits the number of children in the care of one adult. Others have minimal standards, permitting supervision of large groups of children by one caretaker. Further, many states have few requirements for staff training and the level of training can affect the quality of care (Morgan et al., 1986). Most states have public health laws and regulations relative to communicable diseases. Violation of these may constitute a presumption of or evidence of negligence. Stevenson and colleagues (1986) suggest that difficulty would arise in attempts to assess liability at a children's center unless there were repeated violations of health standards. However, the adequacy of staff response to situations "once an infectious disease has been diagnosed is where the greater area of potential liability lies" (p. 645). Failure to maintain adequate health standards, follow appropriate reporting procedures, notify families in a timely fashion, notify staff, and follow recommendations of public health officials may be cause for legal action.

LIBEL AND SLANDER

Defamation of character involves communication of inaccurate information in which the reputation of a third party is harmed. This harm must be to a degree that others are deterred from associating with the person about whom negative comments have been made (VanBiervliet and Sheldon-Wildgen, 1981). If false material is orally communicated, a *slander suit* may ensue. If untruthful material is communicated in writing or through photographs, a *libel suit* may ensue. Likelihood of slander or libel suits associated with communicable diseases and young children does not seem great. However, it seems wise to caution staff concerning comments about colleagues, children, or families who may have a communicable disease or who may be carriers of a communicable disease. False statements regarding a child or child's family and communicable diseases could have negative consequences for the center or staff member or both. This seems particularly important where a communicable disease is associated with sexual activity, intravenous drug abuse, or hygienic standards. These are sensitive value-laden issues and inaccurate statements could provoke a strong response.

INVASION OF PRIVACY AND CONFIDENTIALITY

To receive official recognition by a state education agency or receive funding from federal education agencies, preschool programs must comply with federal, state, and local statutes and regulations regarding confidentiality. The Family Educational Rights and Privacy Act of 1974, also known as the Buckley-Pell Amendment (Turnbull, 1986), assures confidentiality of any "personally identifiable data, information, and records" (p.200). Further, a breach of this trust may lead to a "violation of privacy" suit (VanBiervliet and Sheldon-Wildgen, 1981). Violation of privacy is a disclosure of private information which may be factual, but is of a personal nature and not considered appropriate for public disclosure. This may have implications for information related to communicable diseases.

While program administrators have a responsibility to protect a client's confidentiality, there is also an obligation to protect others from possible infection. When experiencing an outbreak of a communicable disease at a children's center, it is imperative that other families receive information regarding the possibility of infection. In order to avoid a breach of confidentiality, a general letter (see Figure 6-1) containing a description of any illness involved in an outbreak of a communicable disease at a center should be sent to all families with children enrolled. Information about the illness, its characteristics, modes of transmission, likelihood of infection, and precautionary or treatment measures should be included in the letter (Georgetown University Child Development Center, 1986).

WHAT ARE POTENTIAL CONSEQUENCES OF NEGLIGENCE, MALPRACTICE, SLANDER, LIBEL, AND INVASION OF PRIVACY?

Negligence, malpractice, slander, libel, and invasion of privacy are considered noncriminal acts or *torts*. In tort cases, courts can require the person committing the wrongful act (defendant) to compensate the injured party (plaintiff). This compensation usually takes the form of a cash award. In lieu of, or in addition to, a cash award, the plaintiff may be entitled to a portion of the defendant's assets, such as real estate or bank accounts.

Figure 6-1. Sample letter to be sent to families if there is an outbreak of hepatitis A. (Adapted from Georgetown University Child Development Center [1986]. *Health in day care: A manual for day care providers.* Washington, DC: Author.)

DATE: _____

DEAR PARENT OR GUARDIAN:

A child or staff member in our center has been found to have a viral infection called hepatitis A, to which your child may have been exposed.

INFORMATION ABOUT HEPATITIS A:

What Is It? Hepatitis A is an infection of the liver caused by a virus. It can cause tiredness, fever, lack of appetite, nausea, and jaundice (yellowing of the skin and whites of the eyes, with darkening of the urine). The illness usually lasts 1 to 2 weeks. Young children do not usually become jaundiced, however, and may have only a "flu-like" illness, or nothing at all.

How Do You Get It? The virus lives in the intestines and is passed out of the body in the stools. The virus is microscopic, so you cannot see it. If individuals do not wash their hands well after toileting a child or themselves, or do not wash the child's hands, the virus can be spread to other people, food, drink, or other things. The germs can then be swallowed by another person, multiply in the intestines, and cause illness 2 to 8 weeks later. If a person is exposed (that is, may have swallowed some germs), the illness may be prevented by a shot of immune globulin.

How Is It Diagnosed? Hepatitis A is diagnosed by a blood test.

What Should You Do About Hepatitis A?

1. Be sure everyone in your household washes their hands *after* going to the toilet, or changing a diaper. They must wash the children's hands, too. *These are the most important things to do!* Hands should also be washed before touching food, eating, or feeding.

2. If anyone in your household develops signs of hepatitis A, ask your health care provider to do a blood test and tell us if it is positive.

3. Do any of the items below which are checked off:

_____ Ask your health care provider to give your child a shot of immune globulin. (The immune globulin is usually available free of charge to your physician from your state or local health department.)

_____ Ask your health care provider to give immune globulin shots to the other people in your household.

RESPONSIBILITIES OF EMPLOYERS AND PROGRAM DIRECTORS

Standards and Practices

Employers or program directors are responsible for establishing standards of education or care. Standards are usually defined in policies or procedures manuals which provide written assurances of a particular course of action (Linder, 1983). Program standards should generally be consistent with standards and practices throughout the field (Brown, 1984; Decker and Decker, 1984). If standards or policies at a particular children's center are inconsistent with reasonable and customary standards and practices, possible litigation following the spread of an infectious disease might address potential discrepancies.

Administrators of preschools and day care centers are encouraged to develop center-based standards and policies which are consistent with national standards and practices. With respect to minimizing the risks of spreading infectious diseases, Table 6-1 contains suggestions for policy issues to be addressed by program administrators (Bredekamp, 1986; Brown, 1984; Committee on Early Childhood, Adoption and Dependent Care: American Academy of Pediatrics, 1987).

Model Standards and Practices

Program directors would be wise to be cognizant of nationally accepted standards and practices for the education and care of young children in group settings. Development of consistent center standards is an important prevention measure with respect to communicable diseases. Virtually all national models address health and safety issues. Model standards and practices have been developed by a variety of national and state organizations including the National Association for the Education of Young Children (NAEYC), the American Public Health Association (APHA), and the American Academy of Pediatrics (AAP). Addresses and phone numbers of these organizations can be found in the Appendix.

NAEYC has been proactive in the development of models for early childhood standards and practices. NAEYC supported establishment of the National Academy of Early Childhood Programs (Bredekamp, 1986), a "national, voluntary accreditation system for early childhood centers and schools" (p. iv). This comprehensive accreditation program addresses a variety of components directed at health and safety of staff, children, and the environment. Any center can apply for an accreditation review. Self-study materials are available for preparation prior to a review and technical

Table 6-1. ISSUES FOR POLICY DEVELOPMENT RELATIVE TO LEGAL ISSUES AND COMMUNICABLE DISEASES

Educational practices
  Group size
  Adult-to-child ratio
  Supervisory practices
Environmental quality
  Handwashing procedures
  Disinfecting routines
  Use of disposable products
  Separation of food handlers from caretakers of infants and toddlers
Staff qualifications
  Staff screening
Orientation of personnel
  Health issues
Health of staff and volunteers
  Carrier status
  Immunizations
  Physical evaluation
  Limitations
Health of children
  Carrier status
  Immunizations
  Physical evaluation
  Limitations
Accident and illness reporting
  Emergency procedures
  Procedures for cleaning spills of body fluids
  Accidents
  Illness
  Emergency contacts
Food handling
Confidentiality
  Access to records
Children with special needs
  Problem behaviors
Parent notification in the event of an outbreak

assistance can be obtained. NAEYC's model for accreditation has been reviewed by professionals throughout the field of early childhood education and child care and found to be an excellent mechanism for establishment of standards and practices for day care centers and preschools.

The Committee on Early Childhood, Adoption and Dependent Care of the American Academy of Pediatrics (1987) offers specific suggestions for policies related to health in child care centers. Information regarding policies for staff health appraisals, child illness, exclusion, disease control, and child health records is included in this useful reference manual.

Professionals from the American Public Health Association (APHA) have pursued a collaborative project with the American Academy of Pediatrics (AAP) to develop national health and safety performance standards for out-of-home child care programs (American Public Health Association, in press). Of the ten public health issues addressed in this project, a number are particularly relevant to communicable diseases and group settings for young children, including (1) environmental quality, (2) prevention and control of infectious disease, (3) general health (of children and families), (4) staff health, (5) children with special needs (including children with chronic illness), and (6) health and safety organization and administration. APHA standards should provide guidance for those who strive to minimize the risk of transmitting communicable diseases in group settings for young children.

Confidentiality

As described previously, centers which receive federal support must comply with the Family Educational Rights and Privacy Act (FERPA) of 1974 (Turnbull, 1986). Proprietary or nonprofit day care centers may not be bound by FERPA requirements. However, many states have regulatory requirements for confidentiality. If a child has a communicable disease (e.g., hepatitis A), a center's staff is expected to hold that child's identity in confidence. However, there is also an obligation to provide a safe and healthful environment for all children attending the program. In order to protect the rights of children who are ill while protecting the rights of other children, it is important for administrators to develop careful policies, procedures, and staff training programs covering these issues.

Staff Qualifications

VanBiervliet and Sheldon-Wildgen (1981) cite three basic duties of teachers: (1) provision of adequate supervision, (2) use of good judgment, and (3) proper instruction. These also seem to be reasonable expectations for care providers of young children. Proper training of those who educate and care for young children should address these issues and employers should develop hiring practices which will increase the likelihood of recruiting and retaining staff members who are properly trained in educational methodologies and materials and who demonstrate sound judgment.

Realistically, current social policies and regulations do not support preparation of educators and care providers concerned with programs for young children. Early childhood workers are frequently paid minimum wages, have few benefits, and are unregulated with respect to training (Morgan et al.,

1986). Zigler and Muenchow (1986) report that some states do not even require a high school diploma or orientation training for day care providers.

Training

As noted previously, regulatory practices regarding training of those who care, educate, and care for young children is minimal. Kendall and colleagues (1986) discuss the importance of training with respect to health promotion and disease prevention. If this training was not obtained prior to employment, it is critical that orientation training include this information. The following are issues to consider for training purposes: (1) relationships between child physical health and emotional well-being; (2) prevention, identification, and management of infectious diseases in children; and (3) staff health issues (Kendall et al., 1986). Aronson and Aiken (1980) developed a training model for health advocates in child care programs. This could be adapted for early childhood educators and care providers. Training could also include the use of written materials. For example, materials disseminated by the U. S. Department of Health and Human Services (1984) could be shared for review prior to assumption of child-related activities.

Consultation Related to Health Issues

The APHA and AAP offer information on the use of pediatric health consultants for children's centers (Committee on Early Childhood, Adoption and Dependent Care: American Academy of Pediatrics, 1987; American Public Health Association, in press). As described previously, private pediatricians, public health officials, local health department professionals, pediatric nurse-practitioners, and other health care providers can provide valuable advice and assistance with respect to communicable diseases. Review of health-related policies and procedures, advice regarding signs and symptoms of illness, and parent education materials are but a few of the ways in which a pediatric health care consultant can offer assistance to child care centers. Given the special problems associated with communicable diseases in children's centers, it seems particularly important to have access to health care professionals who can offer timely advice on a variety of issues related to the health of young children, their families, and staff.

Insurance

VanBiervliet and Sheldon-Wildgen (1981) suggest that "adequate insurance coverage has become an absolute necessity for all profit and nonprofit organizations as well as for private citizens" (p. 72). In many states liability insurance is required for educational or child care facilities. The center and some or all employees may be covered under this kind of policy. Professional organizations also offer group policies for participating members (Brown, 1984). It seems unlikely that a children's center or staff member would be the target of litigation related to communicable diseases; however, it is wise to take precautionary measures.

Workers' compensation. Workers' compensation is a benefit for most employees throughout the United States. In some states, organizations with few employees are excluded from mandatory coverage, and three states have elective laws pertaining to workers' compensation. Workers' compensation was designed to provide protection for employees who are injured as a result of a job-related accident. Initially these laws did not recognize job-related illness. Currently all states have specific workers' compensation provisions for occupational diseases such as silicosis and radiation-related diseases. Infectious diseases have received little attention. Pursuit of workers' compensation due to infection in the workplace warrants exploration by employers and employees. However, workers' compensation coverage in the event of an outbreak of a communicable disease is uncertain until precedents can be fully established (Stevenson et al., 1986).

RESPONSIBILITIES OF EMPLOYEES

Preparation

"Many states have virtually no requirements for staff training" (Zigler and Muenchow, 1986). Although prior training may not be required, employees at children's centers have an obligation as a substitute parent, or one who serves in loco parentis, to be adequately prepared for duties related to the care of children. Training in child development, early childhood education, and child care is available in some secondary schools, vocational centers, junior colleges, colleges, universities, and other programs. Given the low pay of most child care establishments, there is little incentive for those who care for children to pursue costly training related to the development and education of children. However, there are compelling reasons for pursuing education related to child issues. Zigler and Muenchow (1986) report on research which indicates that workers trained in child care were far more attentive to children than those with no specialized training. Also, children who attended centers with trained staff scored higher on standardized tests than peers at centers with untrained workers. If a teacher or child care worker supports the importance of an optimal environment for child development, it is important to have adequate preparation for working with young children.

Knowledge of Policies and Procedures

Teachers and child care workers have an ethical responsibility to be familiar with center policies and procedures. For example, policies related to disclosure of carrier status could affect specific job assignments. It might be necessary to assign those who are communicable disease carriers to duties which would not present health hazards. Employees who are carriers of giardia should not engage in food preparation activities and should be assigned to care for older children.

Insurance

No one likes to consider the possibility of being sued. As mentioned in the introductory paragraph, lawsuits have become fairly commonplace in contemporary culture (VanBiervliet and Sheldon-Wildgen, 1981). Insurance policies written for children's centers may involve individual coverage; however, the amount of coverage may not be enough to provide adequate individual protection. Teachers and child care workers should be encouraged to consider additional protection, if appropriate. Most professional organizations now provide group insurance rates for liability policies as well as other kinds of health, disability, and life insurance.

Continuing Education

Continuing education is an important aspect of any career. Children's centers may have regularly scheduled inservice training sessions or provide support for staff to attend local, regional, or national educational conferences. Formal presentations and workshops at conferences provide a wealth of information. Presentations and collegiality at professional conferences provide an opportunity for updates regarding research and innovative practices. Journals, textbooks, and materials prepared by professional organizations also serve as sources of information regarding current trends and issues in the education and care of young children.

There are a variety of postsecondary educational opportunities. Many junior colleges, colleges, and universities offer undergraduate or graduate programs in early childhood education or related fields. To keep up with research, methods, and materials, or to qualify for pay increases, many choose to pursue a degree from an accredited higher education facility.

Any of these strategies can be employed to gain further training and education in issues related to young children. Health issues should be incorporated into training sessions or classes. It is often possible to request special topics for inservice sessions, or ask for inclusion of health issues in course-work designed to prepare early childhood educators.

Participating in professional organizations can provide ongoing training. Professional journals, meetings, and newsletters provide forums for information exchange related to young children. The benefits of membership and participation in professional organizations are multiple, but the ongoing educational aspect of membership is probably one of the most important benefits.

Another particularly important aspect of professional organizations that relates to young children and communicable diseases is the power of organizations to lobby for statutory and regulatory changes which promote the health of children and adults who work with young children. A variety of organizations advocate national, state, and local regulatory sanctions which would require implementation of policies and procedures designed to minimize the risks of transmitting communicable diseases in group settings for young children. The importance of this collaborative effort cannot be stressed too strongly. Zigler and Muenchow (1986) report the need for model federal regulatory practices or policies which support (1) smaller group sizes for young children, (2) better staff-to-child ratios in children's centers, (3) specialized training in child development and hygiene, and (4) strategies for recruitment and retention of qualified service providers.

Health

Given the susceptibility (Klein, 1986) of young children to infection, common sense would dictate that teachers and other care providers should strive to maintain good health. Contact with adults free of disease serves to decrease opportunities for infection in young children. Development of healthy habits related to nutrition, rest, recreation, and relationships appears to be positively associated with increased resistance to illness (McCubbin, Cauble, and Patterson, 1982).

SUMMARY

Although it would be difficult to anticipate all possible events related to communicable diseases and the legal issues which might arise, planning is critical to prevent or minimize potential problems. Program leaders should consider a range of legal issues and prepare policies and inservice programs which address those of concern. State laws, regulations, and standard practices should be considered when developing policies and procedures. When these are substandard in comparison with national practices, the prudent administrator will meet and exceed minimal requirements in order to provide a safe healthy environment for young children and to minimize liability exposure.

SUGGESTED READING

Bredekamp, S. (Ed.). (1986). *Developmentally appropriate practice*. Washington, DC: National Association for the Education of Young Children.

Brown, J. F. (1984). *Administering programs for young children*. Washington, DC: National Association for the Education of Young Children.

Committee on Early Childhood, Adoption and Dependent Care: American Academy of Pediatrics (1987). *Health in day care: A manual for health professionals*. Elk Grove Village, IL: American Academy of Pediatrics.

Linder, T. W. (1983). *Early childhood special education: Program development and administration*. Baltimore, MD: Paul H. Brookes.

References

American Public Health Association (in press). *Model standards: A guide for community preventive health services*. Washington, DC: Author.

Andersen, R. D., Bale, J. F., Blackman, J. A., and Murph, J. R. (1986). *Infections in children: A sourcebook for educators and child care providers*. Rockville, MD: Aspen.

Aronson, S. S., and Aiken, L. S. (1980). Compliance of child care programs with health and safety standards: Impact of program evaluation and advocate training. *Pediatrics, 65*, 318–325.

Aronson, S. S., and Osterholm, M. T. (1984, December). Prevention and management of infectious diseases in child care. *Child Care Information Exchange*, pp. 8–10.

Black, H. C. (1979). *Black's law dictionary*. St. Paul, MN: West.

Bredekamp, S. (Ed.). (1986). *Developmentally appropriate practice*. Washington, DC: National Association for the Education of Young Children.

Bricker, D. D. (1986). *Early education of at-risk and handicapped infants, toddlers, and preschool children*. Glenview, IL: Scott, Foresman.

Brown, J. F. (Ed.). (1984). *Administering programs for young children*. Washington, DC: National Association for the Education of Young Children.

Centers for Disease Control (1985). Prevalence of cytomegalovirus excretion from children in five day-care centers—Alabama. *Morbidity and Mortality Weekly Report, 34*, 49–51.

Centers for Disease Control (1985). Education and foster care of children infected with human T-lymphotrophic virus type III/lymphadenopathy–associated virus. *Morbidity and Mortality Weekly Report, 34*, 518–521.

Child Day Care Infectious Disease Study Group (1984). Public health considerations of infectious diseases in child day care centers. *Journal of Pediatrics, 105*, 683–686.

Children's Defense Fund (1986). *A children's defense budget*. Washington, DC: Author.

Committee on Early Childhood, Adoption and Dependent Care: American Academy of Pediatrics (1987). *Health in day care: A manual for health professionals*. Elk Grove Village, IL: American Academy of Pediatrics.

Committee on Infectious Diseases: American Academy of Pediatrics (1987). Health guidelines for the attendance in day-care and foster care settings of children infected with human immunodeficiency virus. *Pediatrics, 79*, 466–471.

Crosson, F. J., Black, S. B., Trumpp, C. E., Grossman, M., Lé, C. T., and Yeager, A. S. (1986). Infections in day-care centers. *Current Problems in Pediatrics, 16*, 122–184.

Decker, C. A., and Decker, J. R. (1984). *Planning and administering early childhood programs* (3rd ed.). Columbus, OH: Charles E. Merrill.

Evans, A. S. (Ed.). (1982). *Viral Infections of Humans*. New York: Plenum.

Fields, B. N. (Ed.). (1985). *Virology*. New York: Raven Press.

Fleming, D. W., Cochi, S. L., Hull, H. F., Helgerson, S. D., Cundiff, D. R., and Broome, C. V. (1986). Prevention of *Haemophilus influenzae* type b infections in day care: A public health perspective. *Reviews of Infectious Diseases, 8*, 568–571.

Ford–Jones, E. L., Kim, M. M., Yaffe, B. A., Ford–Jones, A. E. A., Abelson, W. H., Issenman, R. M., and Gold, R. (1987). Infectious diseases in day–care centres: Minimizing the risk. *Canadian Medical Journal, 137*, 105–107.

Fraas, C. J. (1986). *Preschool programs for the education of handicapped children: Background, issues, and federal policy options* (CRS Report No. 86-55EPW). Washington, DC: Congressional Research Service, Library of Congress.

Georgetown University Child Development Center. (1986). *Health in day care: A manual for day care providers*. Washington, DC: Author.

Gehrz, R. C. (1984). *CMV: Diagnosis, prevention, and treatment*. St. Paul, MN: Children's Hospital of St. Paul.

Gong, V., and Rudnick, N. (Eds.). (1987). *AIDS, facts and issues*. New Brunswick, NJ: Rutgers University Press.

Gross, P. A., and Levine, J. F. (1987). Immunizations: Part I. *Roche Handbook of Differential Diagnosis, 6* (13).

Guralnick, M. J. (1978). *Early intervention and the integration of handicapped and nonhandicapped children*. Baltimore, MD: University Park Press.

Hadler, S. C., and McFarland, L. (1986). Hepatitis in day care centers: Epidemiology and prevention. *Reviews of Infectious Diseases, 8*, 548–557.

Hollingsworth, J. (1986). *Unspeakable acts*. New York: Congdon & Weed.

Ilg, F. L., and Ames, L. B. (1955). *Child behavior: From birth to ten*. New York: Harper & Row.

Interview with Sergio Stagno: Isolation precautions for patients with cytomegalovirus infection (1982). *Pediatric Infectious Disease, 1*, 145–147.

Jordan, A. E. (1986). The unresolved child care dilemma: Care for the acutely ill child. *Reviews of Infectious Diseases, 8*, 626–630.

Kendall, E. A., Aronson, S. S., Goldberg, S., and Smith, H. (1986). Training for child day care staff and for licensing and regulatory personnel in the prevention of infectious disease transmission. *Reviews of Infectious Diseases, 8*, 651–656.

Klein, J. O. (1986). Infectious diseases in day care. *Reviews of Infectious Diseases, 8*, 521–526.

Linder, T. W. (1983). *Early childhood special education: Program development and administration*. Baltimore, MD: Paul H. Brookes.

MacDonald, K. L., Danila, R. N., and Osterholm, M. T. (1986). Infection with human T-lymphotrophic virus type III/lymphadenopathy-associated virus: Considerations for transmission in the day care setting. *Reviews of Infectious Diseases, 8*, 606–612.

Mann, J. M., and Chin, J. (1988). AIDS: A global perspective. *New England Journal of Medicine, 319*, 302–303.

McCubbin, H. I., Cauble, A. E., and Patterson, J. M. (Eds.). (1982). *Family stress, coping, and social support*. Springfield, IL: Charles C Thomas.

Morgan, G. G., Stevenson, C. S., Fiene, R., and Stephens, K. O. (1986). Gaps and excesses in the regulation of child day care: Report of a panel. *Reviews of Infectious Diseases, 8*, 634–643.

Morrison, G. S. (1988). *Early childhood education today* (4th ed.). Columbus, OH: Charles E. Merrill.

Pass, F. P., Hutto, C., Ricks, R., and Cloud, G. A. (1986). Increased rate of cytomegalovirus infection among parents of children attending day-care centers. *New England Journal of Medicine, 314*, 1414–1417.

Payne, C. (Ed.). (1983). *Programs to strengthen families: A resource guide*. New Haven, CT: Yale Bush Center in Child Development and Social Policy.

Petersen, N. J., and Bressler, G. K. (1986). Design and modification of the day care environment. *Reviews of Infectious Diseases, 8,* 618–621.

Riesman, D. (1935). *The story of medicine in the Middle Ages.* New York: Paul B. Hoeber.

Shapiro, E. D., Kuritsky, J., and Potter, J. (1986). Policies for the exclusion of ill children from group day care: An unresolved dilemma. *Reviews of Infectious Diseases, 8,* 622–625.

Silverman, B. K., and Waddell, A. (Eds.). (1987). *Report of the Surgeon General's workshop on children with HIV infection and their families* (U.S. Dept. of Health and Human Services publication No. HRS-D-MC 87-1). Washington, DC: U. S. Government Printing Office.

Sleator, E. K. (1983). *Infectious diseases in day care.* Urbana, IL: Clearinghouse on Elementary and Early Childhood Education, University of Illinois.

Starr, P. (1982). *The social transformation of American medicine.* New York:Basic Books.

Stedman's medical dictionary (24th ed.). (1982). Baltimore, MD: Williams & Wilkins.

Stevenson, C. S., Sterne, G. S., and Stephens, K. O. (1986). Liability for infectious diseases in day care: Legal and practical considerations. *Reviews of Infectious Diseases, 8,* 644–647.

Turnbull, H. R. (1986). *Free appropriate public education: The law and children with disabilities.* Denver, CO: Love.

U. S. Department of Health and Human Services, Public Health Service, and Centers for Disease Control (1984). *What you can do to stop disease in the child day care center: A kit for child day care directors* (U. S. Dept. of Health and Human Services Publication No. 017-023-00172-8). Washington, DC: U. S. Government Printing Office.

VanBiervliet, A., and Sheldon-Wildgen, J. (1981). *Liability issues in community–based programs: Legal principles, problem areas, and recommendations.* Baltimore, MD: Paul H. Brookes.

Wehrle, P. F., and Franklin, H. T. (Eds.). (1981). *Communicable and infectious diseases* (9th ed.). St. Louis: C. V. Mosby.

Weiner, R., and Hume, M. (1987). *And education for all: Public policy and handicapped children.* Alexandria, VA: Capitol Publications.

Zigler, E., and Muenchow, S. (1986). Infectious diseases in day care: Parallels between psychologically and physically healthy care. *Reviews of Infectious Diseases, 8,* 514–520.

Appendix

Resources

There are many local, state, and national resources available for further information about communicable diseases and young children. This list is not comprehensive, but serves as a guide to select professional organizations, reference books for adults, and books for use in children's educational programs.

ORGANIZATIONS

American Academy of Pediatrics (AAP)
P.O. Box 927, 141 Northwest Point Blvd.
Elk Grove Village, IL 60009-0927
(312) 228-5005

The academy serves as an advocacy and educational group with respect to children and their health. Special committees and study groups have been formed to focus on infectious disease issues as they pertain to young children in group settings. Educational materials have been developed for use with health care workers, educators, and parents.

American Public Health Association (APHA)
1015 15th St., NW
Washington, DC 20005
(202) 789-5600

APHA is active in education relating to public health concerns of children. Currently, APHA is involved with efforts to set standards related to health and safety issues for out-of-home care of children.

Association for the Care of Children's Health (ACCH)
3615 Wisconsin Ave., NW
Washington, DC 20016
(202) 244-1801

For 20 years, ACCH has been in the forefront of advances in pediatric health care via advocacy, education, and research. ACCH is concerned with psychosocial and developmental needs of children and families in health care settings. Publications and products include:

- When your child has a life-threatening illness (1983)

- The chronically ill child and family in the community (1982)

- Preparing children and families for health care encounters (1980)

Members of ACCH are entitled to reduced registration fees for the annual conference and local meetings, regular issues of *Children's Health Care* (the official journal of ACCH), the ACCH bimonthly newsletter, and timely notification of newly developed ACCH publications.

Centers for Disease Control
U.S. Department of Health and Human Services
Atlanta, GA 30333
(404) 639-3311
The Centers for Disease Control (CDC) has a variety of publications related to the management of communicable diseases in group settings for young children. An interagency group has been formed to explore issues related to child care and communicable diseases.

Child Care Information Exchange
P. O. Box 2890
Redmond, WA 98073
(206) 882-1066
The Child Care Information Exchange publishes a bimonthly journal designed primarily for child care directors. A variety of issues are addressed in the journal, including curriculum, legislative initiatives, child custody conflicts, technology applications in early childhood, and health guidelines for child care centers. Susan Aronson, M.D., a consultant on pediatric infectious diseases and child care, is a frequent contributor to this publication.

Children's Defense Fund (CDF)
122 C St., NW
Washington, DC 20001
(202) 628-8787
CDF is a national organization dedicated to lobbying and educational activities on behalf of children. CDF is especially concerned with issues affecting poor, minority, and handicapped children. CDF gathers relevant information and statistics and coordinates legislative efforts regarding issues affecting children.

National Association for the Education of Young
Children (NAEYC)
1834 Connecticut Ave., NW
Washington, DC 20009
(202) 232-8777
  NAEYC has a variety of publications related to young children in group settings. NAEYC's recommendations for standards in group settings of young
children includes a section on hygiene and offers guidelines for health-
related practices. To obtain a listing of publications offered through NAEYC,
call or write their national headquarters.

PUBLICATIONS FOR ADULTS

Andersen, R. D., Bale, J. F., Blackman, J. A., and Murph, J. R. (1986). *Infections in children: A sourcebook for educators and child care providers.* Rockville, MD: Aspen.
  *This text offers a variety of information regarding infection in children. Common childhood illnesses,
their modes of transmission, and preventive techniques are presented. The appendix contains information
sheets suitable for use with parents, and other materials appropriate for educational and child care settings.*

California State Department of Education (1983). *Techniques for preventing the spread of infectious
diseases.* Sacramento, CA: Author.
  *The California State Department of Education offers protocols for hand washing, diapering, and class-
room cleanliness. The use of jargon is minimal in this highly readable and informative publication. This
and other relevant publications can be obtained for a small fee from:*
California State Department of Education
P.O. Box 271
Sacramento, CA 95802

Children's Hospital of St. Paul (1984). *CMV: Diagnosis, prevention and treatment.* St. Paul, MN:
Author.
  *Staff of the clinical and research programs at Children's Hospital of St. Paul have been active in the study
of cytomegalovirus (CMV). They have prepared a highly readable, thorough pamphlet related to basic facts
about CMV transmission, CMV and pregnancy, congenital CMV infection, testing for CMV, treatment,
and research. Guidelines and bibliography are also included. This publication would be a valuable addition to the library of any professional concerned with young children and their health. To order, write or call:*
Children's Hospital
345 North Smith Ave.
St. Paul, MN 55102
(612) 298-8835

Committee on Early Childhood, Adoption and Dependent Care: American Academy of Pediatrics. (1987). *Health in day care: A manual for health professionals.* Elk Grove Village, IL: American
Academy of Pediatrics.
  *Selma Deitch, M.D., provided editorial leadership for this informative guide for health professionals,
child care directors, teachers, and parents. Included in this text are guidelines for safe and healthy:*

- *Environments*
- *Child activities*
- *Staff practices*
- *Policies*
- *Diet and food preparation*

There are special sections related to children with developmental disabilities, child abuse, child care regulations, and infectious diseases. This comprehensive manual should be useful to anyone concerned about young children and child care. This text can be ordered from:
American Academy of Pediatrics
P. O. Box 927, 141 Northwest Point Blvd.
Elk Grove Village, IL 60009-0927
(312) 228-5005

Committee on Infectious Diseases: American Academy of Pediatrics (1988). *Report of the committee on infectious diseases* (21st ed.). Elk Grove Village, IL: American Academy of Pediatrics.
   More commonly known as "the red book," this report contains recommendations developed by the American Academy of Pediatrics' Committee on Infectious Diseases, in conjunction with the Centers for Disease Control, the Food and Drug Administration, the National Institutes of Health, and the Canadian Paediatric Society. Suggested vaccination schedules and summaries of infectious diseases are the mainstay of this standard reference. In recent years, sections related to children in out-of-home care and management of children who have been sexually abused have been added. Although this may not be needed as a reference book in every setting involving groups of young children, program directors and teachers may want to consult this text at the local library periodically. To order, write or phone:
American Academy of Pediatrics
P. O. Box 927, 141 Northwest Point Blvd.
Elk Grove Village, IL 60009-0927
(312) 228-5005

Council for Exceptional Children (1986). *Report of the Council for Exceptional Children's task force on policy issues relating to the management of students with communicable diseases.* Reston, VA: Author.
   The Council for Exceptional Children is an international professional organization concerned with handicapped and gifted children and youth. In 1985, a task force, chaired by Dr. Gloria Egnoth of Baltimore County Public Schools in Maryland, examined communicable disease issues related to handicapped children and youth. The task force offers an analysis of issues and policy suggestions for management of students with communicable diseases. A copy can be obtained from:
Council for Exceptional Children
1920 Association Drive
Reston, VA 22091-1589
(703) 620-3660

Crosson, F. J., Black, S. B., Trumpp, C. E., Grossman, M., Lé, C. T., and Yeager, A. S. (1986). Infections in day-care centers. *Current Problems in Pediatrics, 16,* 129–184.
   This entire issue was devoted to the problem of infection in child care settings. As described in the foreward, "This well-organized monograph provides information needed to prevent, diagnose, and manage" (p. 125) specific diseases. A comprehensive table is included which lists diseases, their causative organism, the frequency of transmission in day care, the mode of transmission, and appropriate intervention strategies. Copies of this journal can be ordered from:
Year Book Medical Publishers
35 East Wacker Drive
Chicago, IL 60601

Pokorni, J. L., and Kaufmann, R. K. (1986). *Health in day care: A training guide for day care providers.* Washington, DC: Georgetown University Child Development Center.
   Publication of this manual was supported by the Administration of Children, Youth and Families and the U. S. Department of Health and Human Services' Division of Maternal and Child Health. These agencies contracted with the Georgetown University Child Development Center to provide a document which focuses on training related to minimizing the spread of infectious diseases and reducing the incidence of accidents in child care settings. Training activities are outlined for correct hand washing procedures, exclusion guidelines, and routes of transmission for infectious diseases. An accompanying manual, Health in

day care: A manual for day care providers, *can be obtained from the same source and is designed to be used in conjunction with training activities. Manuals can be ordered from:*
Georgetown University Child Development Center
3800 Reservoir Road, NW
Washington, DC 20007
(202) 687-8635

Silverman, B. K. and Waddell, A. (Eds.). (1987). *Report on the Surgeon General's workshop on children with HIV infection and their families* (U.S. Dept. of Health and Human Services publication No. HRS-D-MC 87-1). Washington, DC: U.S.Government Printing Office.
In April 1986, Surgeon General C. Everett Koop convened the third national conference of health care leaders who were concerned about children infected with the human immunodeficiency virus (HIV) and their families. Proceedings include:

- *The global epidemiology of acquired immunodeficiency syndrome (AIDS)*

- *The human immunodeficiency virus (HIV)*

- *Transmission of HIV in the United States*

- *The natural history of pediatric HIV infection*

- *Preventive approaches to HIV transmission*

- *The transmission of HIV through blood products*

- *Supportive care and treatment of pediatric AIDS patients*

- *Legal issues*

- *Current developments and future prospects with respect to development of an AIDS vaccine*
  The information is relatively technical, but provides important information on pediatric AIDS and HIV infection.

Sleator, E. K. (1983). *Infectious diseases in day care.* Urbana, IL: Clearinghouse on Elementary and Early Childhood Education, University of Illinois.
This publication was prepared as an educational tool for those concerned about health issues related to out-of-home care of young children. The author suggests a need for revision of traditional policies of excluding ill children from center-based programs in favor of more progressive, medically sound policies which do not cause undue hardship for working parents with young children. Issues are presented in an orderly, readable format designed for the lay reader.

U. S. Department of Health and Human Services, Public Health Service, and Centers for Disease Control (1984). *What you can do to stop disease in the child day care center: A kit for child day care directors* (U.S. Dept. of Health and Human Services Publication No. 017-023-00172-8). Washington, DC: U. S. Government Printing Office.
This kit was developed to provide accurate information relative to minimizing the spread of communicable diseases in day care centers. It is written in lay language and contains:

- *A handbook for center directors*

- *A handbook for caregivers*

- *A handbook for parents*

- *A handbook containing general information about communicable diseases as a reference for the center*

- *Posters designed to remind caregivers of procedures which can minimize the spread of communicable diseases.*

Specific suggestions for training sessions are contained and materials have been carefully presented in an attractive, readable format which should be useful to anyone interested in young children and their health.

PUBLICATIONS FOR CHILDREN

Bruun, R. D. and Bruun, B. (1982). *The human body.* New York: Random House.
An array of clear illustrations regarding the human body and its workings are provided. Although communicable disease is not addressed as a separate issue, various body systems (e.g., tissues and cells, the digestive, respiratory, and circulatory systems) are described. Accompanying illustrations provide a forum for classroom discussions and reference.

Caselli, G. (1987). *The human body: And how it works.* New York: Grossett & Dunlap.
Body systems are described and illustrated in great detail. This text would be an appropriate reference for 4- and 5-year-old children. Sections on ''interesting facts'' and ''animal-human comparisons'' provide rich material for classroom discussions and curricular units related to science.

Donner, C. (1986). *The magic anatomy book.* New York: W. H. Freeman.
Precocious young children interested in human anatomy and physiology will probably find this book informative. The author tells a fantasy story of two children who become extremely small and embark on a journey through a human body. This text-intensive story could be used at story time, a chapter at a time, or by early readers with an interest in science.

Kaufman, J. (1987). *Joe Kaufman's big book about the human body.* New York: Western.
The colorful illustrations and lively text make this book especially appealing to young children. Although, there is too much information in this text to make it appropriate for story time, it would be a wonderful reference book and a valuable resource for inevitable discussions about the workings of the human body. A section on illness and health is especially pertinent to discussions of communicable diseases.

McGuire, L. (1974). *You: How your body works.* New York: Platt & Munk.
The narrative style of this book makes it an appropriate choice for story time. It is highly readable and has delightful, whimsical illustrations which provide introductory material for young children who are beginning to develop an awareness of their bodies and health issues. Short chapters entitled ''Why do you breathe all the time,'' ''What makes that thumping noise in your chest,'' and ''Taking care of your body'' give brief, basic information on the respiratory and circulatory systems.

Packard, M. (1985). *From head to toes: How your body works.* New York: Simon & Schuster.
Clear, age-appropriate illustrations and text are provided in this book. The section on heart, blood, and circulation offers an explanation of ways in which the human body fights germs and infection. Other sections (e.g., ''stomach, intestines and digestion'') provide a basis for discussions related to communicable diseases.

Index

Accreditation of child care
    programs, 66–67
Acquired defense mechanisms,
    23–24
Acquired immunodeficiency
    syndrome, 7, 37, 43–45, 52
    transmission of, 44–45
Active immunity, 24
Adenoviruses, 16
Administrators of child care
    centers, 66
Admission application, evaluation
    of, 50–51
AIDS. *See* Acquired
    immunodeficiency syndrome
American Academy of Pediatrics,
    44, 48, 50, 52–56, 66–69, 73,
    78, 79
    day care policy of, 48
American Public Health
    Association, 66, 68, 69, 75
Antibody, 11, 22
Antibody testing, 48
Antigen, 11, 21
Arboviruses, 16
Arenaviruses, 16
Association for the Care of
    Children's Health, 79
Asymptomatic infection, 39

Bacilli, 14
Bacteria, 12, 13
    disease-causing, 15
    friendly, 14
    identification of, 4
    life cycle of, 13
    normal, 14–15
Bacteriology, 12
Bacteroides, 14
Band-Aids, 30
Behaviors
    self-help, 30
    social, of young children, 30
Biblical references, 2–3
Birth, acquired immunodeficiency
    syndrome and, 44

Bisexual men, acquired
    immunodeficiency syndrome
    and, 44
Biting, 49
Black death, 3
Bleach, 47
    as disinfectant, 55
Blisters, fever, 39
Blood, transmission of disease and,
    44
Blood cells, white, 43
Blood transmission, 44
Body fluid spills, 58
Breach
    of confidentiality, 64
    of duty, 62
Breast milk, 44
Buboes, 2
Bubonic plague, 3–4
Buckley-Pell Amendment, 64
Building ventilation, 8

Candida, 14
Car pools, 31
Carrier, 11, 13
Causative agents, 37
CDC. *See* Centers for Disease
    Control
Cellular immunity, 23
Centers for Disease Control, 8, 24,
    30, 41, 49, 75, 80
Chickenpox, 16, 18, 37, 39, 52
Child
    acquired immunodeficiency
        syndrome and, 44
    handicapped, 28, 35
    illness in, 29, 31
        day care policy for, 49
    immunity, 29
    learning, 28
    preverbal, 29
Child birth, acquired
    immunodeficiency syndrome
    and, 44